Optics, Retinoscopy, and Refractometry

Second Edition

Al Lens, COMT
Pro-lens Ophthalmic Services
Vancouver, BC

Series Editors:
Janice K. Ledford • Ken Daniels • Robert Campbell

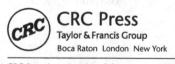

CRC Press
Taylor & Francis Group
Boca Raton London New York

CRC Press is an imprint of the
Taylor & Francis Group, an **informa** business

First published 2006 by SLACK Incorporated

Published 2024 by CRC Press
2385 NW Executive Center Drive, Suite 320, Boca Raton FL 33431

and by CRC Press
4 Park Square, Milton Park, Abingdon, Oxon, OX14 4RN

CRC Press is an imprint of Taylor & Francis Group, LLC

Library of Congress Cataloging-in-Publication Data

Lens, Al.
    Optics, retinoscopy, and refractometry / Al Lens. -- 2nd ed.
      p. ; cm.
    Includes bibliographical references and index.
    ISBN-13: 978-1-55642-748-0 (alk. paper)
    1. Eye--Accommodation and refraction. 2. Retinoscopy. 3. Physio-
logical optics.   I. Title.
    [DNLM: 1. Refractive Errors--diagnosis. 2. Optics. 3. Refracto-
metry--methods. 4. Retinoscopy--methods.   WW 300 L573o 2006]
    RE925.L46 2006
    617.7'55--dc22
                                        2005030167

ISBN: 9781556427480 (pbk)
ISBN: 9781003525462 (ebk)

DOI: 10.1201/9781003525462

Dedication, Second Edition

This book is dedicated to my wife Sheila and daughters Bridgette and Meagan.

Dedication, First Edition

This book is dedicated to my beloved parents, Henry and Sheila.

Contents

Acknowledgments, Second Edition

My family continues to put up with my workaholic tendencies, and for that I am grateful. To all the ingenious people who find ways to improve on technology in the ophthalmic field, I truly admire you. There are too many to name, and I would not even know who many are, but I am glad these people exist so that we can take better care of our patients and help countless people see better than ever thought possible.

Acknowledgments, First Edition

It is a pleasure to acknowledge the people who have made a contribution to my ability to write this book. First, without the generosity of Dr. Howard Gimbel, I would not have had an opportunity to work in ophthalmology. Judy Gimbel encouraged me to write *The Ophthalmic Assisting Guide*, followed several years later by the second edition. I am indebted to my family—my wife, Sheila, and daughters, Bridgette and Meagan—who have been supportive during all the days and nights I have spent writing. And, of course, my appreciation to Jan Ledford, the editor of this wonderful series, who has been kindly critiquing my work.

About the Author

Al Lens began his ophthalmic career in 1986 at the Gimbel Eye Centre in Calgary, Alberta, Canada. His keen interest in learning and teaching put him in the position of training ophthalmic assistants. After writing *The Ophthalmic Assistant Guide*, Al began lecturing across North America at various conferences. His teaching has taken him as far away as Saudi Arabia. He is author of *LASIK for Technicians* and coauthor of *Ocular Anatomy and Physiology* and *Cataracts and Glaucoma*. The latter 2 publications are part of *The Basic Bookshelf for Eyecare Professionals Series*.

The Study Icons

The Basic Bookshelf for Eyecare Professionals Series is quality educational material designed for professionals in all branches of eyecare. Because so many of you want to expand your careers, we have made a special effort to include information needed for certification exams. When these study icons appear in the margin of a *Series* book, it is your cue that the material next to the icon (which may be a paragraph or an entire section) is listed as a criteria item for a certification examination. Please use this key to identify the appropriate icon:

OptP   paraoptometric

OptA   paraoptometric assistant

OptT   paraoptometric technician

OphA   ophthalmic assistant

OphT   ophthalmic technician

OphMT   ophthalmic medical technologist

Srg   ophthalmic surgical assisting subspecialty

CL   contact lens registry

Optn   opticianry

RA   retinal angiographer

Chapter 1

Optics

Optn

KEY POINTS

- The two main theories of light travel are the corpuscular theory and the wave theory. It is uncertain which theory is correct, but it seems that light has both properties.

- The speed of light in a vacuum is 186,282 miles per second.

- The two main factors that determine the power of a lens are the index of refraction (IR) and the curvature.

- Light emanating from a light source is always divergent (ie, spreads apart).

- A prism will affect the direction of light but not its vergence.

- Light striking a reflective surface will be reflected at an angle equal to the incoming light.

Optics in ophthalmology can be divided into three components: physical, geometric, and physiologic. Physical optics studies light itself, including the theories of light travel and the electromagnetic spectrum. Geometric optics relates to how light rays are affected by various surfaces and media. Physiologic optics involves the mechanism, psychology, and physiology of vision and seeing.

Physical Optics

There are two main theories regarding light travel: the corpuscular theory and the wave theory (not to be confused with wavefront). According to the corpuscular theory, light energy coming from a light source is like tiny bullets shooting outward in straight lines in all directions. This theory is helpful when trying to understand ray diagrams, real image formation, and reflection by mirrors. The wave theory says that light behaves like a wave as it passes through transparent material. This applies when studying how light is bent by various media. It is uncertain which theory is correct, but it seems that light has features of both properties—corpuscular and wave.

The electromagnetic spectrum encompasses all light energy, ranging from the shortest (cosmic) rays to the longest (radio) waves. Clinical optics includes the spectrum from ultraviolet to infrared. In the middle of the ultraviolet and infrared spectrum is visible light (Figure 1-1). White light is a combination of all the colors while black is the absence of all colors. The pattern of color in visible light follows a certain order according to its wavelength (the distance between the peak of adjacent waves), which is evident when light passes through a prism. A popular mnemonic used to remember the order of the colors from longest (760 nanometers [nm]) to shortest (400 nm) is the "name" Roy G. Biv (red, orange, yellow, green, blue, indigo, and violet). There are numerous reasons for knowing the light spectrum. It helps in understanding:
- Certain clinical tests (such as the red-green duochrome test).
- The range of lasers.
- Color vision deficiencies.

The speed of light in a vacuum is 186,282 miles per second. This speed changes in different media (this is discussed more in the next section). There is only a nominal difference in the speed of light in air vs that in a vacuum, so the speed of light through a vacuum is used in mathematical equations in optics.

Geometric Optics

Light travels in a straight line until its path is bent by a medium. (A medium is a substance that light can pass through, such as gas, liquid, or glass.) Bending of light is called refraction. In optics, the media we usually deal with are lenses of some type. Lenses can cause light to come to a focus (ie, have a focal point). As the strength of the lens increases, the focal point is moved closer to the lens. The distance between the center of a lens and the focal point is known as the focal length (Figure 1-2).

The power of a lens is measured in diopters (D). A 1 D lens will bend parallel light rays to a focal point that is 1 meter (m) from the lens. To put it in a formula, D is equal to the reciprocal of the focal length of the lens (in meters); the formula is $D = 1 \div F$, where D is the dioptric power of the lens, and F is the focal length of the lens (in meters). For example, when parallel light (from a distant source) enters a lens and focuses 2 m away, $D = 1 \div 2 = 0.5$; therefore, the lens is 0.50 D in strength. A lens that focuses parallel light 10 centimeters (cm) (0.10 m) from the lens would be 10.00 D in power $(1 \div 0.1 = 10)$. Table 1-1 shows the focal lengths of various lenses.

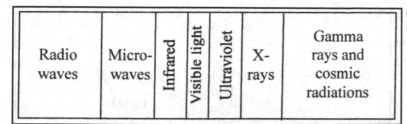

Figure 1-1. The electro-magnetic spectrum.

Radio waves	Micro-waves	Infrared	Visible light	Ultraviolet	X-rays	Gamma rays and cosmic radiations

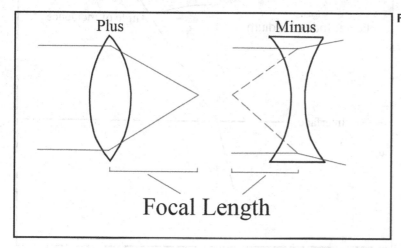

Figure 1-2. Focal length.

Plus   Minus

Focal Length

Table 1-1
Lens Power Compared to Focal Length

Lens Power	Focal Length
0.5 D	2 m (200 cm)
1.0 D	1 m (100 cm)
2.0 D	0.50 m (50 cm)
3.0 D	0.33 m (33 cm)
4.0 D	0.25 m (25 cm)
5.0 D	0.20 m (20 cm)
6.0 D	0.17 m (17 cm)
7.0 D	0.14 m (14 cm)
8.0 D	0.13 m (13 cm)
9.0 D	0.11 m (11 cm)
10.0 D	0.10 m (10 cm)

The focal length of a lens is related to its power. Lenses with shorter focal lengths have higher powers and vice versa. The power of a lens is typically rounded to two decimal places. Also, the sign should always be noted. (Mathematically, numbers are considered positive unless otherwise noted, but this is not the case when speaking of lenses.)

There are two main factors that determine the power of a lens: the index of refraction (IR) of the lens and the curvature. The IR refers to the speed that light can travel through a medium. Mathematically, the IR equals the speed of light in a vacuum divided by the speed of light in the substance. The speed of light in a vacuum is 186,282 miles per second, and the speed of light in water is approximately 140,000 miles per second: $186,282 \div 140,000 = 1.33$ (IR of water). As the IR increases, so does the effect of that medium on light (to bend it more). The speed of light

Figure 1-3. Light passing through an interface of two media. Light bends toward the normal line in the medium with the higher IR.

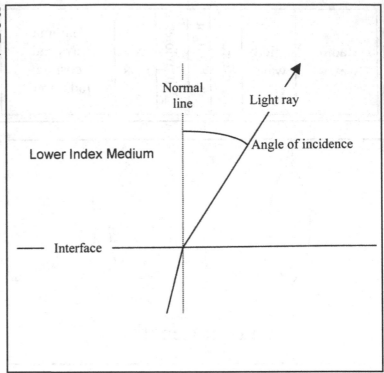

through a medium is inversely proportionate to the IR (ie, the higher the IR, the slower light travels through that medium). The optical structures of the eye have different IRs (if all the structures had the same IR, the eye would be a single, thick lens). Materials to make spectacle lenses are available in various IRs. (The cost for the lens tends to rise along with its IR.)

The curvature of a lens also affects the lens' power. Light entering a medium perpendicular to its surface will not change direction but will travel through the medium in a straight line. The light that enters the medium is known as the incident ray (Figure 1-3). The angle of incidence is the angle formed between the incoming light ray and an imaginary line extended perpendicular to the surface of the medium. If light is bent by the medium, the amount of bending is measured as the angle of refraction (also measured perpendicular to the surface). The light emerging from the medium is the emergent ray. The direction of the emergent ray forms the emergent angle and is measured perpendicular to the surface of the medium.

When the front and back surfaces of the medium are parallel to each other (like a pane of glass), the emergent angle will equal the incident angle, and the focus will not be affected (Figure 1-4). A medium with refractive power (ie, one that refracts light) does not have parallel surfaces—at least one surface will be curved. Lenses used for ophthalmic purposes may be spherical (same power in all meridians) or cylindrical (having two primary meridians—one with maximum refractive power and one with no power). Ophthalmic lenses can be either convex (thicker in the center than at the edges) or concave (thicker at the edges than at the center). All lens design depends on the constant relationship of the incident angle, angle of refraction, and the IR.

It is possible to determine the angle of refraction if the IR of both media is known along with the angle of incidence. This is done by using Snell's law (the basic law of refraction): sine of the angle of incidence ÷ sine of the angle of refraction (written as $n \sin i = n' \sin i'$ where n = IR of the first medium, n' = the IR of the second medium, i = angle of incidence, and i' = the angle of refraction).

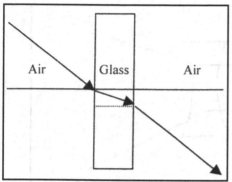

Figure 1-4. Light passing through glass at an oblique angle. Angle of emergent ray is the same as incoming ray.

This formula is commonly used by individuals who design lenses. If you are interested in increasing your understanding of how the direction of light can be calculated, follow the example below.

Example:

n = 1.00 (IR of air)

n' = 1.33 (IR of water)

i = 40

i' = ?

This example is written as (1.0) (sin 40) = (1.33) (sin i') which can also be rearranged to— (1.0) (sin 40)/1.33 = sin i'. Unless you really like algebra, it is best to use a scientific calculator to do the sine calculations. In case you do not have said calculator handy, the sine of 40 is 0.643. Therefore, the problem is rewritten as: sin i' = (1.0) (0.643) ÷ 1.33 = 0.483. Using a scientific calculator, 0.483 is the sine of 28.9 degrees; therefore, the angle of refraction is 28.9 degrees.

Light emanating from a light source is always divergent (ie, rays spread apart as they travel away from the source). If the source is more than 20 feet (6 m) away, then the light can be considered to have parallel rays (although they are still very slightly divergent). Light traveling through a lens will have its vergence (the angles of the rays of light in relation to each other) affected. This effect will depend on the properties of the lens. Parallel light entering a minus-powered lens will become divergent (negative vergence or spreading apart of the light rays), whereas a plus-powered lens causes convergence (positive vergence or coming together of light rays toward a focus) (Figure 1-5).

Plus-powered lenses are used to correct hyperopia (farsightedness) and cause magnification of the image. Minus-powered lenses correct myopia (nearsightedness) and cause minification. High plus-powered lenses will cause a noticeable pincushion effect (looking at a door, the top and bottom of the door looks wider than the middle). High minus-powered lenses create a barrel distortion (the middle of the door appears wider than the top and bottom). Aspheric lenses that have less power in the periphery can be used to decrease these distortions.

Light passing through a lens produces an image. Sometimes this image is real, other times it is virtual. First, one should understand that *object* rays exist only on the incoming side of an optical system, and *image* rays exist only on the outgoing side. (An optical system is a lens, or a combination of more than one lens, and the surrounding media, usually air.) When the image is on the same side as the outgoing rays, it is called a *real* image. *Virtual* images appear on the *same side* of the lens as the incoming rays. Generally speaking, real images can be formed on a screen, whereas virtual images cannot.

When parallel rays (from 20 feet or more away) enter a plus-powered lens, a real, inverted image is created on the opposite side of the lens (Figure 1-6a). However, since a minus-powered

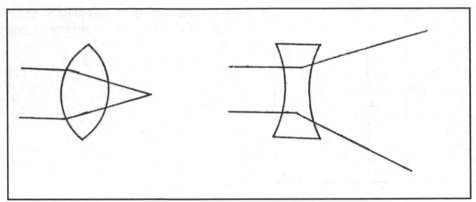

Figure 1-5. Light bent throug minus lens. (Drawing by Holly Hess. Reprinted with permission from Ledford J. *Exercises in Refractometry.* Thorofare, NJ: SLACK Incorporated; 1990.)

Figure 1-6a. A +5.00-D lens converges parallel light and creates a real inverted image 20 cm from the lens.

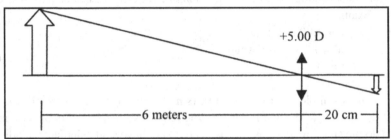

Figure 1-6b. A -5.00-D lens creates a virtual erect image at 20 cm in front of the lens.

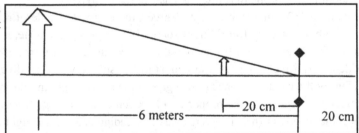

lens causes light to diverge, its focal point is in front of the lens (on the same side as the object), thereby producing a virtual, upright image (Figure 1-6b). The distance between the center of the lens and the focal point is the focal distance.

Of course, light does not always come from a distant object. However, it is still possible to determine the location of the image formation using this formula: U + P = V, where U is the vergence of the object rays (in D), P is the power of the lens (in D), and V is the vergence of the image rays (in D).

Example:

The object (U) is located 0.5 m from the lens. The lens has a power (P) of +6.00. Where does the image lie (V)?

Solution:

Remember that light emanating from an object (the source) always spreads out. We speak of this as negative vergence, or divergence.

Since the object is located 0.5 m from the lens, it has a vergence power of -2.0 (1 ÷ 0.5); therefore, U = -2.0. Using the formula, U + P = V, -2.0 + 6.0 = +4.0. Since D = 1.0 ÷ F (the formula

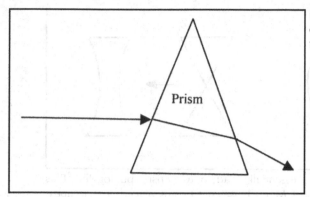

Figure 1-7. Light is bent toward the base of a prism. The image is deviated toward the apex.

mentioned earlier for determining the diopter power), the focal point for this scenario is 1.0 ÷ 4.0 or 0.25 m (25 cm) from the lens.

Lenses

Prisms

A prism will affect the direction of light but not its vergence. Light traveling through a prism will be bent toward the base (thickest part) of the prism. The image will appear toward the apex (thinnest part) of the prism (Figure 1-7). Prisms are commonly used to correct double vision caused by strabismus (misalignment of the eyes). Although the strabismus will still be present, the prism will shift the image to coincide with the visual axis of the eye. Prisms are also used to measure strabismus.

The unit of measure for prisms is a prism diopter. The power of a prism is determined by the amount of deviation of light (in centimeters) that occurs at 1 m. One prism D will deviate light 1 cm at 1.0 m, 2.0 prism D will deviate 2.0 cm at 1.0 m, etc.

The following formula can be used to determine to power of a prism: prism diopters = deviation (in centimeters) ÷ distance (in meters) from the prism.

Example of calculating prism power: If light is deviated 3.25 cm at a distance of 2.0 m from the prism, what is the power of the prism? According to the formula, prism power is equal to the amount of deviation in centimeters (in this case, 3.25 cm) divided by the distance from lens in meters (in our example, 2.0 m). Therefore, the prism power equals 3.25 ÷ 2.0, or 1.625.

Spherical Lenses

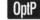

A lens that has the same curvature and power in all directions is called a spherical lens. This type of lens causes light to either converge (bend toward a focal point) or diverge (spread apart). Plus-powered spherical lenses have positive vergence power, causing parallel light to converge. Minus-powered lenses have negative vergence, which causes light to diverge. The point within the lens that has no effect on light is called the optical center. This coincides with the thickest point of a plus lens or the thinnest point of a minus lens. It is not necessarily the geometric center of the lens.

Spherical lenses can be considered to be a combination of prisms. A plus-powered lens is similar to placing prisms base to base. Placing prisms apex to apex simulates a minus-powered lens (Figure 1-8). Understanding that light is bent toward the base of a prism explains why plus and minus lenses refract light as they do. (See "Induced Prism" for more details).

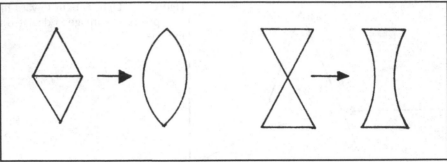

Figure 1-8. Plus and minus lenses are essentially made of two prisms put together. Plus lenses are prisms placed base to base. Minus lenses are prisms placed apex to apex. (Drawing by Holly Hess. Reprinted with permission from Ledford J. *Exercises in Refractometry*. Thorofare, NJ: SLACK Incorporated; 1990.)

Figure 1-9. The power of a cylinder is 90 degrees away from its axis.

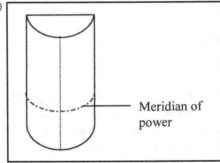

Meridian of power

Cylinders

Cylindrical lenses create a focal *line* instead of a focal point. This focal line is parallel to the axis of the cylinder, but the greatest power of the lens lies perpendicular to its axis in what is called the meridian of power (Figure 1-9). Cylindrical lenses are used to correct astigmatism (explained later in this chapter, in the section on Physiologic Optics, under "Refractive Errors"). A spherocylindrical combination (sphere and cylinder lenses together) produces a situation in which the two focal lines are perpendicular to each other (one line parallel to the cylinder axis and the other focal line along the meridian of power of the cylinder) (Figure 1-10). The space between the two lines is known as Sturm's interval. The conical shape produced by the light rays

within Sturm's interval is called Sturm's conoid. In the middle of the conoid is the circle of least confusion—the point at which vision is clearest while astigmatism is present.

Cardinal Points

Any optical element (ie, anything that alters the vergence of light) has two focal points. For a plus lens, the first focal point from a distant object is in front of the lens, (on the same side as the object) and the second focal point is behind the lens (Figure 1-11). The opposite is true for minus lenses. Complex lens systems (ie, a combination of two or more lenses) have two principal planes. These planes, which replace the front and back surface of a single lens, allow the observer to consider the complex lens system as a single, thin lens. The primary principal plane represents the location of the single lens for incoming rays while the secondary principal plane is where the rays of light leaving the optical system may be considered to have been refracted by a

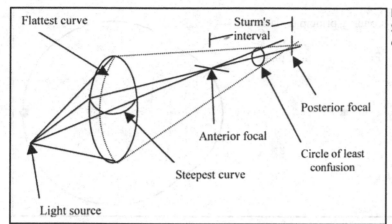

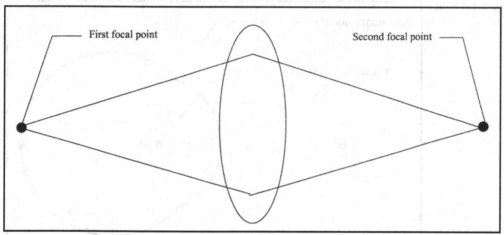

Figure 1-10. Conoid of Sturm formed by a sphero-cylindrical lens.

Flattest curve

Sturm's interval

Posterior focal

Anterior focal

Circle of least confusion

Steepest curve

Light source

First focal point

Second focal point

Figure 1-11. Focal points.

single lens (Figure 1-12). Lastly are the two nodal points. Light entering the optical system is directed toward the primary nodal point and leaves as though it passed through the secondary nodal point without changing its direction (Figure 1-13).

Transposition

Refractors come equipped with plus or minus cylinders but not both. At times, it is desirable to compare a spherocylindrical combination of one type of cylinder with the other. For example, a patient shows you a prescription written in minus cylinder format and wants to know if it compares favorably with one written in plus cylinder. The process of changing a measurement or prescription from one cylinder power to the other is called transposition.

Transposing is a three-step process. First, algebraically add the cylinder to the sphere to calculate the new sphere. (Quick algebra refresher: if the signs are the same, add the two numbers together and keep the sign; if the signs are different, subtract the smaller number from the larger, and keep the sign of the larger number.) Second, the sign of the cylinder is changed. Third, the axis is changed by 90 degrees (but cannot exceed 180 degrees—if the original axis exceeds 90 degrees, then subtract 90 from the original axis).

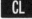

Figure 1-12. Principal planes.

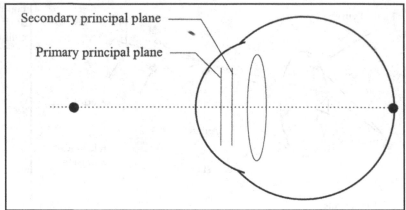

Secondary principal plane

Primary principal plane

Figure 1-13. Nodal points.

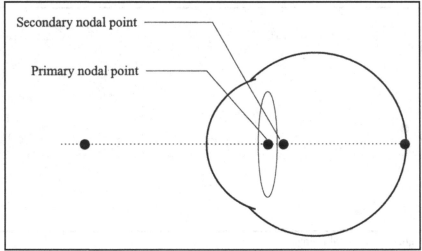

Secondary nodal point

Primary nodal point

For example, to transpose +3.50 -1.50 x 95 to plus cylinder, the cylinder is algebraically added to the sphere [+3.50 + (-1.50)]. This gives us a new sphere value of +2.00. The sign of the cylinder is changed from minus to plus, becoming +1.50. The axis is changed by 90 degrees (the original axis exceeds 90, so use 95 – 90). The new axis is 05. Thus, the plus cylinder equivalent of +3.50 -1.50 x 95 is +2.00 +1.50 x 05.

Spherical Equivalent

When one needs to know the average of a spherocylindrical combination, the spherical equivalent (SE) needs to be calculated. To do this, simply algebraically add 50% (or half) of the cylinder to the sphere, and then disregard the cylindrical values. The SE will be the same whether plus- or minus cylinder format is used. For example, the SE of +3.50 -1.50 x 95 is +2.75. This is calculated by adding -0.75 (-1.50 x 0.5) to +3.50. If the plus cylinder format is used (+2.00 +1.50 x 0.5), the result will be the same, +2.00 + (+1.50 x 0.5) = +2.75. SE is often used in contact lens fitting.

Induced Prism

When light does not pass through the optical center of a lens (the point where there is no change in vergence of light), prismatic effect is induced. The amount of prism induced can be

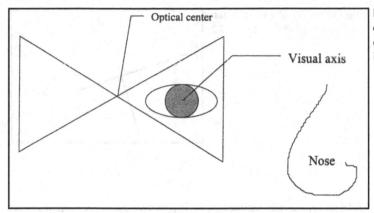

Figure 1-14. A minus-powered lens with optical center dislocated outward, resulting in induced base-in prism.

determined using Prentice's rule (induced prism = decentration [in centimeters] x lens power [in diopters]). This is helpful for determining the amount of induced prism when the optical center of a lens is not aligned with the patient's visual axis. It is helpful to calculate the induced prism when a lens is made with the optical center in the wrong position, when prism is desired in moderate- to high-powered lenses, or when determining if anisometropia (difference in refractive error of the two eyes) will cause problems as the patient looks through the periphery of a lens. Just 1 D of vertical prism can cause diplopia and/or the patient to complain of discomfort. Base-out prism is more easily tolerated than base-in due to a person's ability to converge.

Consider the following example: A patient's interpupillary distance (the distance between the center of the two pupils) is 68 mm; the glasses' pupillary distance (the distance between the optical centers of the two lenses) is 60 mm. In this example, the distance from the center of the bridge of the nose to the center of each pupil is 34 mm, but it is only 30 mm to the optical center of each lens. If the power of each lens is +8.00 D, how much prism is induced for each lens?

Solution: We know that the optical center is 4 mm nasal to the patient's visual axis in each lens, and the power of the lens is +8.00. Prentice's rule states that the induced prism is equal to the decentration in centimeters (in this case 4 mm or 0.4 cm) multiplied by the lens power (in our example, +8.00). Therefore, the induced prism = 0.4 x 8.00 = 3.2 prism D.

The next step is determining the direction of the prism base (the direction in which light will be deviated). Plus-powered lenses induce prism with the base in the same direction as the decentration. For example, if the optical center is decentered nasally, base-in prism is induced; if the optical center is decentered upward, base-up prism is induced. The opposite is true for minus-powered lenses (Figure 1-14).

One last consideration in regard to Prentice's rule: cylinder power needs to be added to the sphere power if the cylinder axis is perpendicular (or nearly perpendicular) to the direction of decentration. This means that if the optical center is decentered in or out, the cylinder power must be considered when the cylinder axis is located vertically; if the optical center is decentered up or down, then the cylinder power is added to the sphere when the cylinder axis is located horizontally. Fifty percent of the cylinder power should be added when the axis is oblique (roughly 45 degrees). Example: the optical center is 5 mm temporal (away from the nose) in a lens measuring -7.00 -3.00 x 90. Since the cylinder axis is perpendicular to the direction of decentration, the cylinder power is added to the sphere (-3.00 is added to -7.00) for a total of -10.00. Using Prentice's rule, induced prism = 0.5 x 10.00 = 5.0 prism D.

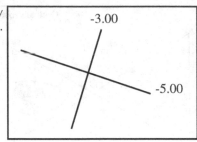

Figure 1-15. Optical cross showing the power of each primary meridian of spherocylindrical combination of -3.00 -2.00 x 72.

The Optical Cross

The powers of a spherocylindrical lens combination can be illustrated using an optical cross. The power of the two primary meridians is labeled on the cross, with its lines representing the location of each meridian. When labeling an optical cross, one must remember that the power of a cylindrical lens is 90 degrees away from its axis. For example, if the cylinder axis is at 80 degrees, its maximal power is 90 degrees away at 170 degrees. This meridian (170 degrees) will reflect the power of the cylinder.

An optical cross will appear the same whether plus or minus cylinder is used. The cross is helpful when using certain formulas such as Prentice's rule (to determine induced prism in any given meridian) and other situations, such as determining the type of astigmatism present (simple, mixed, or compound).

The mathematics involved in an optical cross are simple addition and subtraction. The sphere power is recorded along the line representing the cylinder's axis (ie, the cylinder axis as represented by the prescription or on the refractor). Then, the cylinder power is algebraically added to the sphere power, and this value is recorded along the opposite line (opposite because, as indicated above, its power is 90 degrees away from the meridian). For example, -3.00 -2.00 x 72 can be plotted on optical cross with -3.00 along the 72-degree axis and -5.00 (-2.00 power of cylinder is added to the -3.00 sphere power) along the 162-degree axis (Figure 1-15). The optical cross would appear exactly the same using the plus cylinder equivalent (-5.00 +2.00 x 162).

It is also helpful if you are able to read an optical cross. Determining which meridian represents the sphere will depend on whether you want a plus cylinder result or a minus cylinder result. If you work with plus cylinders, the sphere power is the least plus power (or the most minus power). Vice versa for minus cylinders; the sphere is the most plus (or least minus). The cylinder power is the difference between the two powers on the optical cross. The cylinder axis is along the same axis as the meridian that is labeled with the sphere power.

For example, an optical cross with +7.00 on the line at 90 degrees and +10.00 on the 180 degrees line is interpreted as follows: plus cylinder users would choose the least plus power for the sphere (+7.00), then determine the cylinder power as +3.00 (the difference between +7.00 and +10.00) and the cylinder axis at 90 degrees (that of the sphere). The result: +7.00 + 3.00 x 090. Minus cylinder users would choose the most plus power for the sphere (+10.00), then determine the cylinder power as -3.00 (the difference between +10.00 and +7.00) and the cylinder axis is at 180 degrees (Figure 1-16). The result: +10.00 – 3.00 x 180.

Reflection

When light strikes a reflective surface, it will be reflected at an angle equal to the angle of the incoming light. In other words, the angle of incidence will equal the angle of reflection (law of

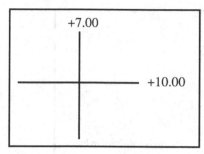

Figure 1-16. Optical cross. Plus cylinder notation: +7.00 +3.00 x 90. Minus cylinder notation: +10.00 -3.00 x 180.

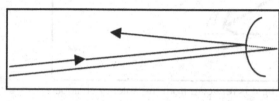

Figure 1-17. Convex mirror creates negative vergence.

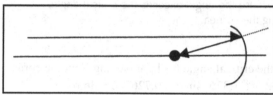

Figure 1-18. Concave mirror creates positive vergence.

reflection). Plane (flat) mirrors do not affect the vergence of light. Convex mirrors add negative vergence, which means they have negative power (Figure 1-17). Convex mirrors will minimize an image. This type of mirror is commonly seen on automobiles (with a warning that states "objects are larger than they appear"). Concave mirrors add positive vergence and, therefore, have positive power (Figure 1-18). These mirrors magnify images. An example of the advantage of this is a shaving mirror.

To determine the power of a mirror, use this formula: power = 2 ÷ radius of curvature (in meters) of the mirror. For example, if the radius of curvature of a convex mirror is 75 mm, what is the power of the mirror? The power is equal to 2 ÷ radius of curvature in meters. Therefore, the power of the mirror = 2 ÷ 0.075 (75 mm = 0.075 m) = 26.67 D. Since it is a convex mirror, it has negative vergence and would be recorded as -26.67 D.

Sometimes, light cannot exit a medium due to a phenomenon known as total internal reflection. This phenomenon prevents us from seeing the anterior chamber angle of the eye without the use of a contact lens, such as the gonio lens (Figure 1-19). Total internal reflection occurs when light moves from a higher index medium to a lower index medium and the *critical angle* is exceeded. Instead of passing into the lower index medium, light is reflected. Think of riding a bicycle alongside a curb and that the curb represents the "jump" to a lower IR than the road; if you ride close to the curb and then try to "jump the curb," you would discover that the "critical angle" has been exceeded, and the wheel would simply be "reflected" back onto the road. However, if you change your angle of approach so that the wheel of the bicycle is approximately 60 degrees to the curb, the bicycle would likely ride up over the curb. This would be like changing the angle of the light to allow it to escape the medium.

The critical angle is dependent on the ratio of the IRs of the two media. To determine the critical angle, we can use the formula: sin c = n' ÷ n, where c = the critical angle, n = the IR of the medium that contains the light, and n' = the IR of the surrounding medium. For example, the IR

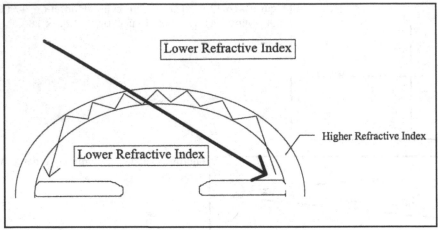

Figure 1-19. Total internal reflection: as light is reflected from the anterior chamber angle, it enters the cornea (higher IR). Because the angle exceeds the critical angle, the light is reflected back instead of exiting the cornea.

of the cornea = 1.376 and the IR of air = 1.00; the critical angle for light passing from the cornea to air would be calculated as follows: $\sin c = 1.00 \div 1.376$; $\sin c = 0.7267$; $c = 46.61$.

Physiologic Optics

The eye is a compound lens system consisting primarily of the cornea and crystalline lens surfaces. The power of this lens system and the axial length of the eye determine the refractive error of an eye. To help explain the optical system of the eye, the schematic eye was developed to indicate the optical constants. The most popular schematic eye is the one developed by Gullstrand (Figure 1-20). (It should be understood, however, that very few real eyes would duplicate the measurements noted in the schematic eye.)

The Schematic Eye

Cornea

According to Gullstrand, the human cornea has a IR of 1.376. The average radius of curvature of the central anterior surface is 7.7 mm, and the posterior surface is 6.8 mm. The radius of curvature refers to the measurement from the center of a circle to its edge; in the case of the cornea, an imaginary circle is created with a curve that is continuous with that of the area being measured (Figure 1-21). The radius of curvature of the cornea translates into a refractive power of +48.83 D on the anterior surface and -5.88 D on the posterior surface. The posterior surface has a negative value because light travels from a higher IR (the cornea's IR is 1.376) to a lower IR (aqueous humor in the anterior chamber has a IR of 1.336). Thus, the total refracting power of the cornea is +42.95 (or +48.83 - 5.88).

The normal cornea is not spherical in shape; it is aspherical. (The term aspheric means "not spherical"; that is, it changes shape or radius of curvature over the entire surface.) The peripheral cornea is flatter (larger radius of curvature) than the central cornea. This aspherical design helps reduce aberration (blurred or distorted image quality) since light passing through the periphery of a spherical lens is bent more than light traveling through the central portion of the same lens.

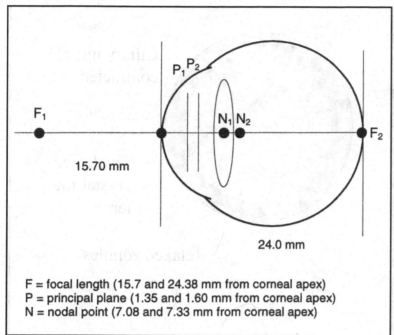

Figure 1-20. Schematic eye.

F = focal length (15.7 and 24.38 mm from corneal apex)
P = principal plane (1.35 and 1.60 mm from corneal apex)
N = nodal point (7.08 and 7.33 mm from corneal apex)

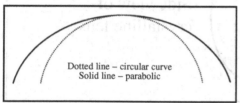

Figure 1-21. Circular and parabolic curves.

Dotted line – circular curve
Solid line – parabolic

Pupil

The pupil is analogous to the aperture (diaphragm) of a camera lens. A larger depth of focus is achieved with a smaller aperture (pupil). Depth of focus refers to the range that is in focus without changing the focus of the lens. The "ideal" pupil size for good quality vision at any distance is between 2 and 5 mm. A pupil that is smaller than 2 mm can cause diffraction (formation of light and dark fringes) to occur. When a pupil expands beyond 5 mm, spherical aberration (blurred image quality) may be noticeable due to the physical optical qualities of the cornea (which tends to bend light more toward its periphery despite its aspheric design discussed earlier).

Crystalline Lens

The lens of the eye consists of two major sections: the cortex, or outer section, surrounds the core (often referred to as the nucleus), or inner section. The IR of the cortex is 1.386, while the core's IR is 1.406; the overall index is considered to be 1.42. When the lens is in its unaccommodated state (explained in a moment), its power is +19.11 D. The maximum power of the lens is +33.06 D with full accommodation. The anterior radius of curvature is 10.0 mm unaccommodated and 5.33 during maximum accommodation. The radius of curvature of the posterior lens surface is 6.0 mm, decreasing to 5.33 mm during maximum accommodation.

Accommodation increases the focusing power of the eye, usually to focus on a near target. When the eye needs to focus on a near target, the ciliary muscle that surrounds the lens receives

Figure 1-22. Ciliary muscle contracted.

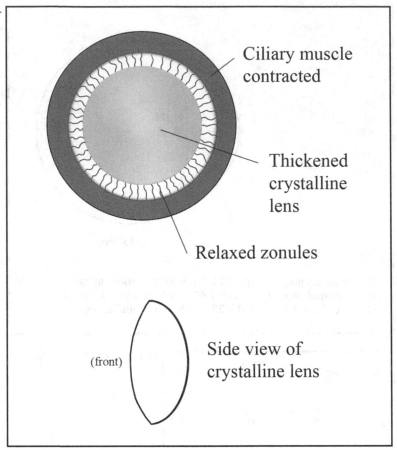

Ciliary muscle contracted

Thickened crystalline lens

Relaxed zonules

(front)

Side view of crystalline lens

a signal to contract. Fine fibers, known as zonules, connect the ciliary muscle to the lens. When the ciliary muscle contracts, the tension on the zonules is reduced, and the lens becomes more powerful (optically speaking) (Figure 1-22). A closer look will reveal that the front surface of the lens bulges in the center, while the periphery remains less curved to limit spherical aberration (discussed in cornea section). The pupil constricts during accommodation to increase depth of field (the area that is in focus without adjusting the accommodation) and further reduce spherical aberration.

Unfortunately, the ability to change the eye's focus diminishes with age. The most common theory for this loss of focusing ability is that there is a continual decrease in elasticity of the lens. This is likely caused by a change in chemical composition when older lens cells are compacted as new lens cells are constantly added throughout a human's life. For the majority of people, the gradual loss of accommodation becomes noticeable around the age of 45 years (Table 1-2). This natural aging phenomenon is known as presbyopia and is treated with reading glasses or bifocals. These plus-powered lenses help to bring the divergent light from a near object closer to parallel (simulating light originating from a distant object). This decreases or eliminates the need for the eye to accommodate.

Axial Length

The axial length (measured from the anterior cornea to the macula) of an average emmetropic eye is 24.4 mm. Assuming that the rest of the eye is average (the lens and cornea are of

Table 1-2
Near Point of Accommodation in Relation to Age

Age	Accommodative Power	Near Point
10 years	14 D	7 cm
20 years	10 D	10 cm
30 years	7 D	14 cm
40 years	4 D	25 cm
50 years	2.5 D	40 cm
60 years	1 D	100 cm

Adapted from Appleton B. Clinical Optics. *Thorofare, NJ: SLACK Incorporated; 1990.*

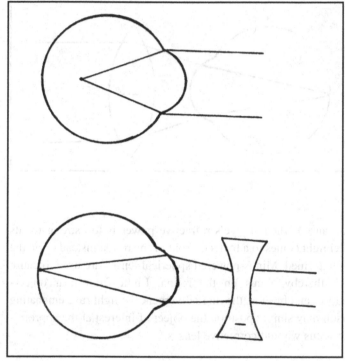

Figure 1-23. Myopia corrected by a minus lens. (Drawing by Holly Hess. Reprinted with permission from Ledford J. *Exercises in Refractometry.* Thorofare, NJ: SLACK Incorporated; 1990.)

average power), approximately 3.0 D of refractive error will be induced for every 1.0 mm change in axial length. If the eye grows larger than normal, myopia (nearsightedness) will be induced (Figure 1-23). Hyperopia is created by an eye that is shorter than normal (Figure 1-24).

Refractive Errors

Objects that are 20 feet or more away emit light with essentially parallel rays. Ideally, these parallel light rays would naturally focus on the retina of the eye without the aid of any lenses or any accommodative effort. This model state is known as emmetropia. Whenever emmetropia is not the case, there is a refractive error, and the image is not focused directly on the retina. Corrective lenses must be worn or accommodation must occur in order to have clear vision. The term ametropia is used to indicate that there is a refractive error (myopia, hyperopia, or astigmatism).

OptA

OphA

CL

OptP

Figure 1-24. Hyperopia corrected by a plus lens. (Drawing by Holly Hess. Reprinted with permission from Ledford J. *Exercises in Refractometry.* Thorofare, NJ: SLACK Incorporated; 1990.)

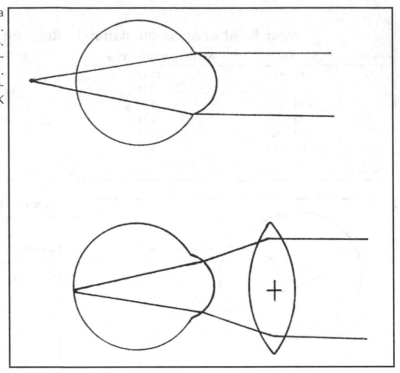

Myopia

Myopia, or nearsightedness, is caused when an eye's refractive power is too strong for its axial length. This means that parallel light comes to a focus in front of the retina instead of on the retina, where a clear image would be formed. Minus-powered spherical lenses are used to cause the parallel light to diverge and, thereby, focus on the retina. Light from near objects naturally has divergent rays—the closer an object is, the more divergent the light rays emanating from it. Therefore, the myopic person may simply position the object of interest at the appropriate (near) distance to obtain a clear focus without corrective lenses.

Hyperopia

Hyperopia, or farsightedness, is caused when an eye's unaccommodated refractive power is insufficient for its axial length. Parallel light is not focused adequately by the lens system of the eye and fails to come to a focus before it reaches the retina. (Theoretically, the light would come to a focus behind the eye.) Plus-powered lenses, or the eye's own accommodation, are used to cause light to focus on the retina.

Hyperopia can be divided into three parts: absolute, manifest, and latent hyperopia. Absolute hyperopia is the amount of hyperopia that cannot be overcome by accommodation; this is measured by the minimum amount of plus sphere that produces best vision. In other words, the patient would require at least this power of lens to see clearly. Manifest hyperopia is represented by the maximum power of plus sphere lens that the patient would accept without compromising his or her vision. Latent hyperopia can only be revealed through the use of cycloplegic eyedrops (used to paralyze accommodation); this is the amount of plus sphere measured above the manifest hyperopia. Example: A hyperope who sees 20/40 uncorrected may require +1.00 sphere to see 20/20 (this means the patient has 1.00 D of absolute hyperopia); this same patient may accept up to +2.50 sphere while still maintaining 20/20 vision (therefore, there are 2.50 D of manifest hyperopia); after cycloplegic drops are used, the patient requires an *additional* +1.50 sphere to see 20/20, for a total of +4.00 (this represents +1.50 D of latent hyperopia, and 4.00 D of *total* hyperopia).

Astigmatism

Astigmatism, in most cases, is caused by an irregularly shaped cornea. If there is regular corneal astigmatism, one meridian of the cornea is the flattest and perpendicular (ie, 90 degrees away) to this is the steepest meridian. This means that light rays passing through the cornea do not focus at a point; rather, there are two focal points, and the image is not clear. Regular astigmatism is entirely correctable with cylindrical lenses, which focus light in a linear fashion and can, thus, be aligned to match the meridian of the astigmatism.

`OptP`

Regular astigmatism can be named according to the location of the greatest refractive power of the eye. Astigmatism can be with-the-rule, against-the-rule, or oblique. With-the-rule astigmatism has the greatest refractive power of the eye in the vertical meridian (ie, minus cylinder axis is at or near 180 degrees, or plus cylinder axis is at or near 90 degrees). Against-the-rule astigmatism has the greatest refractive power in the horizontal meridian (ie, minus cylinder axis is at or near 90 degrees, and plus cylinder axis is at or near 180 degrees). Oblique astigmatism indicates that the greatest refractive power is more than 15 degrees from the horizontal or vertical axis (ie, minus or plus cylinder axis is between 15 and 75 degrees or 105 and 165 degrees).

Another way of classifying astigmatism is by the location of the focal lines within the eye. These classifications are simple, compound, and mixed (Figure 1-25). Simple astigmatism indicates that one focal line is on the retina while the other is either in front of the retina (simple myopic astigmatism) or behind the retina (simple hyperopic astigmatism). Compound astigmatism exists when both focal lines are located either in front of the retina (compound myopic astigmatism) or behind the retina (compound hyperopic astigmatism). When one focal line is in front of the retina and one is behind, mixed astigmatism is present.

Irregular astigmatism is where the flat and steep meridians are not 90 degrees away from each other; this is common in eyes that have suffered trauma. This type of astigmatism cannot be fully corrected with cylindrical lenses. The crystalline lens may also have astigmatism (lenticular astigmatism), which may add to or subtract from the astigmatism in the cornea.

If the axis of the lenticular astigmatism is similar to that of the corneal astigmatism, the total astigmatism would be the sum of the lenticular and corneal astigmatism. Conversely, if the axis of the lenticular astigmatism is perpendicular to that of the cornea, the difference between the two would make up the total astigmatism. Measuring the lenticular astigmatism is done by comparing the corneal astigmatism (from keratometry values) to the refractive amount (the total cylindrical value that provides sharpest vision). If the refractive and corneal values match, there is no lenticular astigmatism. If the refractive amount is higher than the keratometry reading indicates, lenticular astigmatism is present in the same axis. When the keratometry readings show a higher amount of astigmatism than that recorded with refractometry, it is assumed that there is lenticular astigmatism in the opposite axis (90 degrees away).

Retinal Image Size

`OphT`

The size of the image on the retina is typically the same in each eye. When wearing spectacles (and to a lesser degree, contact lenses), myopes will see a smaller image than an emmetrope. Conversely, a hyperope tends to see a larger image. This variation in image size rarely poses a problem unless there is a difference in refractive error between the two eyes (anisometropia).

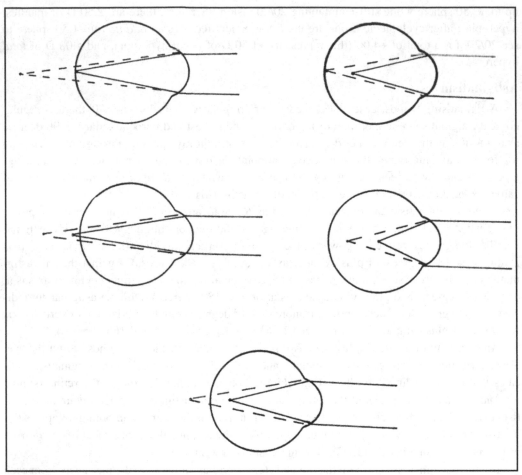

Figure 1-25. (A) Simple hyperopic astigmatism; (B), (E) simple myopic astigmatism; (C) compound hyperopic astigmatism; (D) compound myopic astigmatism; (E) mixed astigmatism. (Drawings by Holly Hess. Reprinted with permission from Ledford J. *Exercises in Refractometry.* Thorofare, NJ: SLACK Incorporated; 1990.)

Small amounts of anisometropia are usually well tolerated. However, when the difference exceeds 3.00 D, there is the potential for a noticeable difference in image size (aniseikonia). Contact lenses are often used in such cases, since the lens is in contact with the eye and there is minimal effect on retinal image size. If contact lenses cannot be worn, the power of one (or both) of the spectacle lenses may have to be altered to lessen the aniseikonia.

According to Knapp's rule, no aniseikonia will result if the refractive error is due only to axial length and corrective lenses are positioned 15 mm in front of the eye, regardless of the refractive error. Knowing this rule may help to increase the success of new spectacles; however, in reality, there are few situations where it can be applied because aniseikonia is rarely caused by axial length alone.

The Optics of Refractive Surgery

There is more than one way to eliminate focusing problems caused by refractive errors in the eye. The old standard of spectacles is still the most common, but refractive surgery is growing in popularity every year. We will take a look at how each type of refractive surgery affects the focus of light coming into the eye.

The Cornea and Refractive Surgery

The cornea is usually uninvolved in most refractive error problems; it is the length of the eye that is responsible for the majority of myopia and hyperopia. Despite this, the cornea is the structure of the eye most commonly altered to reduce or eliminate one's dependency on corrective lenses. It makes some sense because the cornea is responsible for two-thirds of the eye's focusing ability. The average cornea has approximately 43.00 D of focusing power. Even high myopes and high hyperopes will typically have corneas close to that average.

The typical cornea is prolate in shape. That is, the central curvature is steeper than the peripheral curvature. This is good optical design because we know that light coming through a spherical lens will be bent more in the periphery of the lens than the center. By gradually flattening the lens (or cornea) toward the periphery, we produce better quality optics.

A quick look back to the 1980s reveals that radial keratotomy (RK) was the first popular refractive surgery. This procedure involved making radial incisions in the cornea, done freehand by the surgeon, and could correct low to moderate amounts of myopia. The weakening caused by the incisions allowed the peripheral cornea to bulge forward, and a relative flattening of the central cornea would occur. Astigmatic keratotomy (AK) was added to the arsenal shortly thereafter; transverse incisions were made in the cornea in the axis that matched the minus cylinder correction. This caused selective flattening in the desired axis to reduce or eliminate the astigmatism.

Later in the same decade, the excimer laser was introduced to ophthalmology. It was met with much resistance at first because it involved altering the "sacred" central cornea. With RK and AK, the scarring occurred in the periphery and was thought to be of little concern. The concept of removing tissue from the center of the cornea was unthinkable. Thankfully, some people believed it was possible to do this safely.

The excimer laser uses ultraviolet light (wavelength: 193 nm) to reshape the cornea. Rather than relying on altering the structural integrity of the cornea, the laser sculpts a new shape into the cornea by removing stromal cells. Whether the procedure is photorefractive keratectomy (PRK), laser assisted in-situ keratomileusis (LASIK), laser epithelial keratomileusis (LASEK), or epithelial laser assisted in-situ keratomileusis (epi-LASIK or E-LASIK), the end result is the same. The ultimate goal is to eliminate any aberration occurring in the eye, but at the very least, it should reduce or eliminate the lower order aberrations – the same focusing problems that glasses are used to correct.

Surgical Correction of Refractive Errors

For myopia, the intent of corneal refractive surgery is to flatten the cornea, thereby reducing its focusing capabilities. To do this, the excimer laser is programmed to expose more laser light to the center of the cornea (removing more tissue) than to the periphery. Higher amounts of myopic correction, however, will cause the cornea to become oblate – steeper in the periphery than in the center. This less-than-perfect situation can result in loss of contrast sensitivity and night vision problems like glare and halos around lights.

Hyperopia has always proven to be a bit more difficult to correct. While the treatment zone for myopia can be as small as 5 mm (but usually is 6 mm or greater), the procedure for hyperopia requires a larger treatment zone around 9 mm or larger. Smaller treatment zones typically result in regression. To increase the steepness of the cornea to augment the eye's focusing power, a doughnut-like impression is made in the cornea. Tissue is removed from the peripheral cornea while the central cornea remains untouched by the laser. Only mild to moderate amounts of hyperopia can be permanently corrected with laser surgery.

Astigmatism can also be reduced with the excimer laser. Smaller amounts of astigmatism can be eliminated with an ovoid-shaped pattern. Larger amounts, over 3.00 D or so, are often corrected using a cross-cylinder approach: minus cylinder treated in one axis and plus cylinder treated in the opposite axis. The cross-cylinder technique is aimed at limiting any loss of contrast or night vision effects that the smaller ovoid pattern can induce. Before the cross-cylinder approach was possible, many patients who had surgery for high amounts of astigmatism complained of decreased quality of vision. This was mostly due to the narrow side of the ovoid being about 4.5 mm across, far smaller than the average pupil in dim light. Thus, when the pupil dilates, light entering through the uncorrected area of the cornea reaches the retina. This unfocused light causes a halo and/or starburst effect around light sources.

Presbyopia plagues virtually everyone sometime beginning in their 40s. Laser companies have been fervently trying to find a way to eliminate the need for reading glasses. At the time of this writing, a couple of manufacturers have introduced a multifocal treatment that promises to at least reduce the need for the pesky reading glasses. However, it is thought that any time light is divided, contrast sensitivity will be decreased, and other visual problems may develop. This has already been demonstrated with "simultaneous focus" contact lenses where the distant and near focal distances are in focus simultaneously. Multifocal laser eye surgery essentially produces the same effect and, thus, has the same drawbacks. While this is a suitable compromise for some people, for many, it is something they are not willing to tolerate. The new shape of the cornea creates a near-focusing power in the central cornea, and the peripheral cornea will be for distant objects. This causes yet another problem if the pupil constricts within the near segment of the cornea, as now the eye is essentially myopic in that area.

Wavefront

The eye is not the perfect optical system we would like it to be. Even an eye that is emmetropic (no refractive error) can have some subtle optical imperfections. These impurities are known as third or higher order aberrations. In the average eye, higher order aberrations account for about 17% of the total aberration error. Eyes with larger pupils can have noticeably decreased contrast and blurred image edges.

Ophthalmology has enjoyed the utility of corneal topography for many years. The ability to map the curvature of the cornea has made it simpler to understand aberrations caused by an irregularly shaped cornea. Unfortunately, topography is unable to account for internally-caused irregularities. However, recent technology has allowed ophthalmologists to view higher order aberrations using aberrometers.

In the 1970s, adaptive optics was developed to create sharper images from telescopes in space. This science allows the mirrors in the telescopes to be adjusted to account for changes in the atmosphere, thus producing the sharpest image possible. Wavefront analysis observes how a plane of light is focused through an optical system. If no aberrations exist, light from a point image would meet at a single point. Aberrometers can provide detail of the aberrations that exist and lead to the possibility of eliminating them. Ophthalmology has adapted wavefront technology in an effort to create Super Vision – in theory, the wavefront guided excimer laser surgery can produce vision better than 20/20 or even sharper than 20/15. (Some researchers indicate that the human eye would be capable of 20/5 vision if all aberrations were eliminated.)

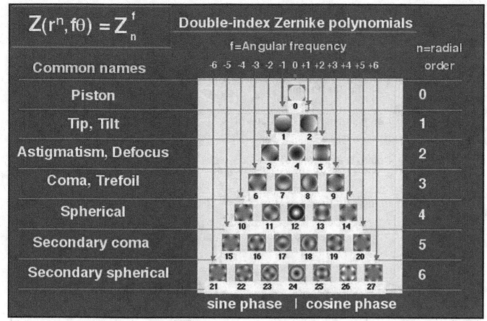

Figure 1-26a. Pictorial directory of Zernike modes used to systemically represent the aberration structure of the eye. (Reprinted in b/w with permission from Krueger, Applegate, MacRae. *Wavefront Customized Visual Correction: The Quest for Super Vision II*. Thorofare, NJ: SLACK Incorporated, 2004.)

It takes complex mathematical formulas to calculate the aberrations that are detected by aberrometers. Frits Zernike won a Nobel prize for physics in 1953 for his demonstration of the phase contrast method, especially for his invention of the phase contrast microscope. His table of polynomials (mathematical expressions) is used extensively in wavefront analysis. Pictorial directories of Zernike modes (Figure 1-26a and Figure 1-26b) demonstrate the shapes of defocus (ie, unfocused images) for the various orders of aberration. The Shack-Hartmann wavefront sensor (Figure 1-27) is used in popular aberrometers to map the aberrations of the eye. The details of such a wavefront-generated map can be read by computers linked to excimer lasers and enable the refractive surgeon to reduce or eliminate some of the higher order aberrations.

Aberrations

There are entire books written on the subject of wavefront analysis and correction, but we will briefly discuss the main defocusing terms here.

Aberrations in general are caused by imperfections in the optical media. Spherical aberrations occur in spherical surfaces when rays that are close to the optical axis (paraxial rays) focus farther from the lens than do the peripheral rays. The farther the points of focus are, the more severe the spherical aberrations.

Astigmatism produces a cone-shaped pattern and is a second order aberration. Light coming into the eye is separated into two lines, typically 90 degrees apart from one another. This is correctable with spectacles or contact lenses.

Coma aberrations are third order aberrations. They result when off-axis rays do not converge on the focal plane. They are not fully correctable with lenses.

Figure 1-26b. Three-dimentional pictorial directory of Zernike modes 0 to 20 (Reprinted in b/w with permission from Krueger, Applegate, MacRae. *Wavefront Customized Visual Correction: The Quest for Super Vision II*. Thorofare, NJ: SLACK Incorporated, 2004).

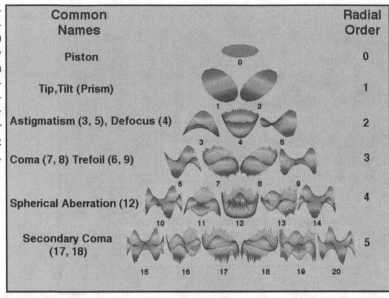

Figure 1-27. Optics of a Shack-Hartman device. A laser beam is expanded, collimated, and focused to a point on the retina. The emerging beam from this point source is focused onto a lenslet array that forms a point pattern that is captured by a video camera. The pattern obtained is compared with that of an aberration-free beam, and again, the wavefront is computed from the displacements of the points from their unaberrated pattern. (Reprinted with permission from Krueger, Applegate, MacRae. *Wavefront Customized Visual Correction: The Quest for Super Vision II*. Thorofare, NJ: SLACK Incorporated, 2004)

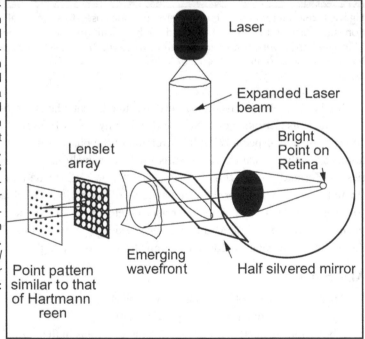

Trefoil aberrations are also in third order of aberrations and consist of three cycles or intervals. Some clinicians refer to trefoil as triangular astigmatism due to its shape being similar to normal astigmatism. The difference is that astigmatism has two axes while trefoil has three.

Quadrafoil is a fourth order aberration with four cycles and is located on the outer part of the Zernike polynomial pyramid. Unlike aberrations that are in the inner aspect of the chart, quadrafoil aberrations tend to be less visually disabling.

Pentafoil is a fifth order aberration with five cycles.

Variabilities in Wavefront

The most challenging aspect of correcting higher order aberrations is probably that they are not constant. They can change with pupil size, variation in the tear film, accommodation, and age.

Individuals with pupils that do not dilate very much will not usually demonstrate a high percentage of third order or higher aberrations. Therefore, wavefront correction is not much of a benefit for them but in most cases, would not be detrimental. Large pupils induce more higher order aberrations and these patients are prime candidates for wavefront correction.

Repeatability of wavefront measurements is relatively high when the tear film is normal but becomes difficult when there is debris or other tear film inconsistencies. It is virtually impossible to obtain three identical wavefront readings, but the variability for most eyes is within a statistically insignificant range.

Accommodation affects the aberrations of the eye to a noticeable degree. Obtaining readings while the eye is accommodating will usually result in different values than when the eye is relaxed. This can be significant if a wavefront correction is being considered and the patient exhibits instrument accommodation (ie, focusing on a near target because the patient mentally knows that the target is within the confines of the relatively small instrument and not 20 feet away). Correcting for aberrations under these circumstances may actually be worse than doing a normal sphero-cylinder correction.

A bigger problem possibly lies with aberrations that change as we age. In theory, we could eliminate all aberrations at the time of surgery, only to have other aberrations chronically appear with each passing year. However, the actual changes appear to be quite subtle from year to year, allowing the benefits of wavefront correction to be enjoyed for an extended period of time.

Wavefront has also allowed for adaptive optics in ophthalmoscopy which has resulted in the ability to examine structures of the human eye in detail never seen before. So, while the attention in wavefront has been in refractive surgery, it has implications on a more clinical level as well.

Intraocular Refractive Surgery

The crystalline lens of the eye cannot be surgically altered unless you consider removing it from the eye an alteration. The lens is contained by a capsular bag. If the thin capsule is punctured or otherwise damaged, a cataract is almost certain to develop, thereby canceling out any benefit that could have possibly been gained by attempting to reshape the lens. So, if we want to alter the eye's focusing ability internally, it is done by placement of an intraocular lens (IOL) instead.

IOLs can be added to the eye without removing the crystalline lens. These lenses are known as phakic IOLs (phakic meaning the eye still has a crystalline lens). The other option is to remove the crystalline lens (called clear lensectomy if there is not a cataract) and replace it with an IOL, resulting in a status known as pseudophakia (artificial lens).

The general rule of thumb used by surgeons is that if accommodation still exists, using phakic IOLs is a better option than removing the natural lens because this maintains the eye's focusing ability. It also implies the patient is relatively young and the mainstream thinking is that it is best to keep the eye as intact as possible for as long as possible.

Removing the crystalline lens of the average eye would result in about 12.00 D of hyperopia at the spectacle plane. This is about 14.00 D at the corneal plane. It takes an IOL of about 23.00 D to achieve emmetropia in an eye that was emmetropic before the crystalline lens was removed.

Myopic eyes would have a lower power implanted or, in some cases, a negative power. Hyperopic eyes need higher IOL powers (and more precise axial length measurements due to the shorter distance being measured). The power of the IOL is calculated by measuring the axial length of the eye (ultrasonically or optically) and the curvature of the cornea (keratometry). A formula is then used to calculate the IOL power.

If the crystalline lens is left intact and a phakic IOL is used, the power of the IOL is calculated primarily on the refractive error of the eye, although other measurements are used (such as keratometry, corneal diameter, and anterior chamber depth).

Prolate IOLs are providing even better vision than the traditional IOLs. The prolate lens has stronger focusing power centrally than peripherally. This is in keeping with the fact that peripheral light rays are bent more than central light rays as they enter a spherical lens. By reducing the power peripherally, the peripheral light does not defocus as much. This is especially noticeable in dim light when the pupil may dilate. Most older people do not have excessively large pupils, so the better quality optics may have limited benefits on the average cataract patient. However, the prolate lens definitely serves a purpose, especially for those who have cataracts earlier in life.

Accommodative IOLs have a unique design that allow the lens to change its effective power and have a range of focus greater than the standard IOL. When the ciliary muscle is stimulated for near acuity, the accommodative IOL's position is adjusted forward. There are a couple of theories on how the accommodative lens is actually moved forward: one theory suggests that there is pressure applied on the lens directly by the ciliary muscle. The second theory indicates that there is increased vitreous pressure caused by the stimulated ciliary muscle, and it is the pressure of the vitreous moving the lens forward. Regardless of how it happens, we know a high plus-powered lens (which most IOLs are) can have its effective power altered by increasing the distance between the lens and the retina. This is much like how a plus-powered spectacle lens is of lesser power than a contact lens, which is closer to the cornea (and retina), to achieve the same effect.

Multifocal IOLs have been around for a couple of decades. A few different designs have been tried with varied success. The current popular multifocal IOL is the AMO Array™ lens, which has multiple zones of focus. The current popular multifocal IOLs are the AMO Array™ lens and the Alcon ReStor lens. These lenses have slightly different methods of producing two primary focus points—one for distance and one for near. 3M had a multifocal lens many years ago that worked on a diffraction principle that used ridges between concentric rings, but these ridges caused halos around lights at night. As with all good things, there are some drawbacks with multifocal IOLs. These drawbacks are mostly related to contrast sensitivity and overall sharpness of vision. Due to the multiple areas of focus, there is some superimposition of focused and unfocused images, which detracts from the overall sharpness and contrast.

Exercises

1. If light from a source more than 20 feet away comes to a focus 20 cm behind a lens, what is the power of the lens?

2. What is the focal length of a -4.50 D lens?

3. Where is the focal point in the above lens (in front of or behind the lens)?

4. Would the image in the above lens be real or virtual?

5. If an object is 33 cm from a +10.00 lens, where is the image (what distance from the lens)?

6. What is the IR of a medium where light travels at 130,000 miles per second?

7. What is the power of a prism that deviates light 4 cm at a distance of 1 m?

8. What is the power of a prism that deviates light 4 cm at a distance of 4 m?

9. Using Prentice's rule, calculate the induced prism: lens power is +8.00 -2.00 x 90 and the optical center of the lens is decentered 3 mm nasally and 2 mm superiorly from the patient's visual axis.

10. What is the power of a concave mirror with a 40 mm radius of curvature?

11. Determine the amount of absolute, manifest, latent, and total hyperopia in the following scenario: the smallest amount of plus-powered lens that achieves best corrected acuity is +1.75 D, but the patient will accept an additional +2.50 D while maintaining best corrected acuity and will take another +1.00 D of plus during the cycloplegic refractometry.

12. Match each type of astigmatism (1 to 5) with its definition (a to e).
    1. Simple myopic astigmatism
    2. Compound hyperopic astigmatism
    3. Mixed astigmatism
    4. Simple hyperopic astigmatism
    5. Compound myopic astigmatism

    a. One focal line in front of the retina and one focal line behind the retina
    b. Both focal lines in front of the retina
    c. One focal line in front of the retina and one focal line on the retina
    d. Both focal lines behind the retina
    e. One focal behind the retina and one focal line on the retina

Answers to Exercises

1. +5.00 D. *Explanation*: Light from a source more than 20 feet away is considered to be parallel and has no vergence power. A focal point of 20 cm (0.2 m) is converted to D (using the formula $D = 1 \div F$); $1 \div 0.2 = 5.00$. The focal point is behind the lens, so it must be plus-powered. Hence, the lens is +5.00 D.

2. 0.22 m or 22 cm. *Explanation*: $D = 1 \div F$; therefore, $4.50 = 1 \div F$; D and F are interchangable in this formula, so $F = 1 \div 4.50 = 0.22$.

3. In front of the lens. *Explanation*: Minus-powered lenses cause light to diverge behind the lens, so the focal point must be in front of the lens.

4. Virtual. *Explanation*: The image is on the same side of the lens as the object and, therefore, cannot be focused on a screen (if a screen is put in front of the lens, the light from the object would be blocked and would not reach the lens—resulting in no image).

5. 14.3 cm behind the lens. *Explanation*: Use the formula $U + P = V$. Light from an object 33 cm away has 3 D of vergence ($D = 1 \div F$). Light from a source is always divergent, so $U = -3.00$ D. $P = +10.00$ (the power of the lens). Using simple math, $-3.00 + (+10.00) = +7.00$. Now, using $D = 1 \div F$ to determine the focal length, $+7.00 = 1 \div F$, or $F = 1 \div 7.00 = 0.143$ m.

6. 1.43. *Explanation:* The speed of light is 186,282 miles per second. The speed of light in the medium is 130,000 miles per second. IR is equal to the speed of light divided by the speed of light in the medium, so $IR = 186,282 \div 130,000 = 1.43$.

7. 4 prism D. *Explanation:* Prism diopters = deviation in centimeters ÷ distance in meters from the prism. Prism diopters = 4 ÷ 1 = 4.

8. 1 prism D. *Explanation:* Prism diopters = deviation in centimeters ÷ distance in meters from the prism. Prism diopters = 4 ÷ 4 = 1.

9. 1.8 base-in prism D and 1.6 base-up prism D. *Explanation:* Prentice's rule is: induced prism = decentration in centimeters x lens power in diopters. Each meridian must be considered separately because of the cylinder power. If the cylinder axis is perpendicular (opposite) to the direction of decentration, the cylinder power must be algebraically added to the sphere. Therefore, for this question, when calculating the horizontally induced prism, the cylinder power must be considered; +8.00 + (-2.00) = +6.00. The horizontal decentration was 3 mm or 0.3 cm. Horizontal induced prism = 6.00 x 0.3 = 1.8 prism D. Plus-powered lenses induce prism with its base in the same direction as the decentration. The decentration was inward, so the horizontally induced prism is 1.8 prism D base-in. In this question, we can disregard the cylinder power for the vertically induced prism (the cylinder axis is parallel to the direction of decentration). Therefore, induced prism = 8.00 x 0.2 = 1.6 prism D. The decentration was upward, so the induced prism base must be up. Hence, 1.6 prism D base-up.

10. +50.00 D. *Explanation:* The formula to be used for calculating the power of a mirror is: 2 ÷ radius of curvature in meters. The radius of curvature is 40 mm or 0.04 m. 2 ÷ 0.04 = 50. A concave mirror has positive vergence, so this mirror has +50.00 D of vergence.

11. 1.75 D of absolute hyperopia, 4.25 D of manifest hyperopia, 1.00 D of latent hyperopia, and 5.25 D of total hyperopia. *Explanation:* The minimum amount of plus to achieve best corrected visual acuity represents the absolute hyperopia (in this case, 1.75 D). The maximum amount of plus accepted while maintaining best corrected visual acuity is the amount of manifest hyperopia (in this case 1.75 + 2.50 = 4.25 D). The difference between the manifest and total hyperopia is the latent hyperopia (in this case 1.00 D). The total amount of plus used during cycloplegic refractometry is the total hyperopia (in this case +4.25 + 1.00 = +5.25 D).

12. 1. = c
    2. = d
    3. = a
    4. = e
    5. = b

Retinoscopy

- There are two basic varieties of streak retinoscopes available—those based on Copeland's design and all the rest.

- A special filament in the bulb of the streak retinoscope creates the linear beam of light.

- For best results, the patient's fixating eye should be fogged to further prevent accommodation.

- The reflex will move in the same direction as the intercept (with-movement) or in the opposite direction (against-movement).

- Plus-powered lenses neutralize with-movement. Minus-powered lenses neutralize against-movement.

- The speed and brightness of the reflex increases as neutralization is approached.

Introduction

Retinoscopy is used to objectively determine the refractive error of an eye. Since no responses are required from the patient, retinoscopy can be performed on a child, a blind person, or even a dog. There are two principal types of retinoscope available—spot and streak. While those who use spot retinoscopes believe their instruments to be superior to streak retinoscopes, we will be describing the technique used in streak retinoscopy. The reason for this selection is due to the immense popularity of the streak retinoscope and not due to any bias on the author's part.

Retinoscopy is an art that is well worth learning. While autorefractors have become quite accurate, an experienced retinoscopist can achieve the same degree of accuracy. Performing retinoscopy also allows the examiner to view the quality of the optical medium of the eye, providing information that the autorefractor cannot. A picture is worth a thousand words—retinoscopy is equivalent to a picture.

Learning the steps involved in retinoscopy is not difficult for most people. Like any art, to become good at retinoscopy requires experience. Many an aspiring retinoscopist reserves practice time for occasions when the trusty autorefractor is unable to provide any hint regarding a particular eye's refractive error. Much to his or her dismay, the inexperienced retinoscopist also fails. This can cause a decrease in the student's confidence, and the retinoscope quickly becomes a dust-collecting light stick. If you want to learn retinoscopy, you must gain experience on eyes with normal media and normal-sized pupils. Once you are proficient in normal eyes, you are ready to begin testing your skills on eyes with small pupils and/or imperfect media.

Equipment

The beginning retinoscopist should have a schematic eye, a refractor, and a retinoscope at his or her disposal. This will allow the student to learn retinoscopy techniques independently and closely simulate the setting that will be encountered when performing retinoscopy on a patient's eye.

Schematic Eye

A retinoscopy schematic eye has an adjustable length to simulate various degrees of hyperopia and myopia. In most cases, the base of the eye can be taped to the headrest of the patient exam chair (Figure 2-1). Astigmatism can be created using cylindrical trial lenses placed in front of the schematic eye (or taped to the back of the refractor). The cylinder should be the opposite format of the refractor being used. That is, if you are using a plus cylinder refractor, a minus-powered cylindrical trial lens is placed in front of the schematic eye.

Each schematic eye has a scale that indicates the amount of myopia or hyperopia that is being simulated. This scale should not be considered to be 100% accurate, and one must remember to factor in the power of the working lens (discussed later in this chapter).

Refractor

A refractor is a device that conveniently encases multiple spherical and cylindrical lenses (Figure 2-2). If a refractor is not available for the retinoscopy student, loose trial lenses can be used with equal accuracy. Many retinoscopy workshops are taught using trial lenses—the only disadvantage is the inconvenience of loose lenses.

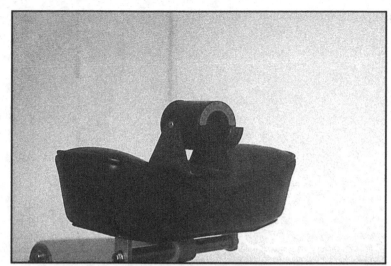

Figure 2-1. Schematic eye affixed to headrest of patient exam chair. This simulates the position of the patient and allows the user to learn retinoscopy with a refractor.

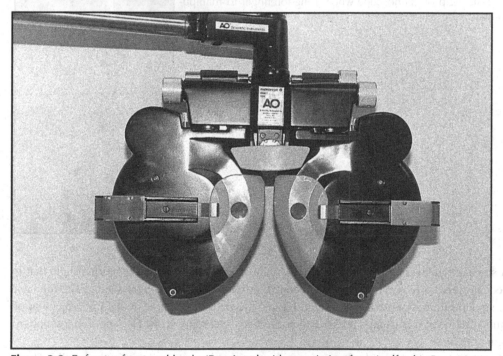

Figure 2-2. Refractor front and back. (Reprinted with permission from Ledford J. *Exercises in Refractometry.* Thorofare, NJ: SLACK Incorporated; 1990.)

Retinoscope

There are two basic varieties of streak retinoscopes available—those based on Copeland's design and all the others. Jack Copeland was the father of streak retinoscopy and spent many years of his life teaching his techniques. Retinoscopes using his design are to be used with the sleeve in the uppermost position (except when using enhancing methods that are discussed later). All other streak retinoscopes are used with the sleeve in the down position. More details about sleeve position are presented in the "Basic Principles" section of this chapter.

Figure 2-3a. Grip on retinoscope when using thumb to manipulate sleeve.

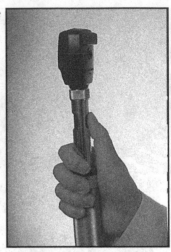

Figure 2-3b. Grip on retinoscope when using forefinger to manipulate sleeve.

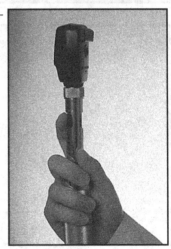

A special filament in the bulb of the streak retinoscope creates the linear beam of light that is emitted. Most bulbs have a filament that is coiled, producing a diffuse light source. The filament in the streak retinoscope's bulb is straight. Hence, the streak of light is actually a projection of the bulb's filament. It is usually possible to convert a streak retinoscope to a spot retinoscope by changing the bulb.

Most retinoscopes sold today operate on a battery that is contained within the handle. These are preferred by most retinoscopists due to the convenience afforded. Some retinoscopes must be plugged into an instrument stand while others can be plugged into a wall receptacle. The power supply only affects the portability of the instrument and the longevity of the available power.

OptT

OphT

Basic Principles

One of the most important aspects of retinoscopy is holding the instrument properly. For convenience and efficiency, a one-handed method for holding the retinoscope must be used. It should be held so that the hand holding the retinoscope can also rotate the sleeve and slide it up and down (Figures 2-3a and 2-3b). Some retinoscopists use their thumb to manipulate the sleeve, while others prefer their forefinger. Develop a style that is most comfortable for you.

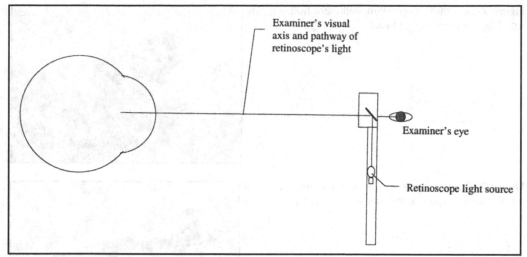

Examiner's visual
axis and pathway of
retinoscope's light

Examiner's eye

Retinoscope light source

Figure 2-4. The pathway of the retinoscope's light and the examiner's visual axis coincide.

The retinoscope should be held with the same hand as the eye that is being examined. Furthermore, the retinoscopist should use the same eye as the hand holding the scope. So, the right hand holds the retinoscope up to the examiner's right eye while he or she is performing retinoscopy on the patient's right eye. This will allow the patient to fixate on a distant target, which is important in order to control accommodation. If the opposite eye is used, the retinoscopist's head tends to block the patient's view of the fixation target.

For best results, the fixating eye should be fogged to further prevent accommodation. Fogging is accomplished by placing a plus-powered sphere before the eye. In the case of myopia, the eye is left uncorrected, which gives the same effect. After the reflex of the first eye has been neutralized (explained below), the working lens (which is a plus lens) should be left in place while doing retinoscopy on the fellow eye. This ensures that the first eye is fogged.

If possible, the retinoscopist should keep both eyes open throughout the exam. Beginning retinoscopists often have difficulty with this task. It may help to limit background light in the room to reduce distractions.

The Reflex and Intercept

Retinoscopy relies on a reflex from inside the eye. If you have seen a photograph of a person who appears to have red pupils, you have seen a reflex of light that is similar to that used in retinoscopy. Red eyes in a photograph are created when the flash is positioned too close to the camera lens; light from the flash illuminates the inside of the eye. This is caught on film because the camera has a viewing angle almost identical to the illumination angle. This same principle is used in retinoscopy design: the observer's viewing angle is the same angle at which the light leaves the retinoscope (Figure 2-4).

Movement of the reflex is often seen when the streak of light from the retinoscope (the intercept which falls on the refractor as well as the patient's iris) is moved. The intention of the retinoscopist is to stop the reflex from moving (known as neutralizing the reflex) by using lenses placed in front of the eye.

The vergence of light from the retinoscope can be adjusted according to the position of the sleeve. When neutralizing the reflex, light rays from the retinoscope should be parallel. This is

Figure 2-5a. Retinoscope with stationary bulb (inserts into base of retinoscope head).

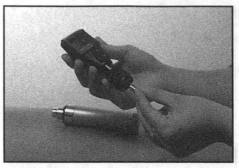

Figure 2-5b. Retinoscope with bulb located on top of handle (bulb moves as the sleeve is moved.)

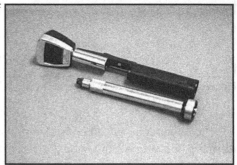

accomplished with a plane-mirror effect. Retinoscopes using Copeland's design have a plane-mirror effect when the sleeve is pushed all the way up (known as the up position). This moves the bulb upward and brings its filament close to a stationary convex lens located toward the top of the retinoscope. The plane-mirror effect of retinoscopes using the alternate design is accomplished when the sleeve is in the down position. These retinoscopes have a stationary bulb; moving the handle down moves the convex lens closer to the bulb (Figures 2-5a and 2-5b).

The correct position of the sleeve for the plane-mirror effect can be determined by holding the retinoscope 33 cm from a flat surface. The position of the sleeve that produces the widest beam of light is the desired position.

Rotating the sleeve will change the axis of the intercept. Some retinoscopes have a separate knob for this purpose. Being able to change the intercept's axis is an integral part of streak retinoscopy. It allows the retinoscopist to analyze the reflex at any axis, which is important when astigmatism is present. (And there is almost always astigmatism present.)

To examine the movement of the reflex, the intercept must be moved perpendicular to its orientation (Figure 2-6). For example, if the intercept is oriented vertically, it is swept from side to side. In this case, the horizontal meridian is the one being scrutinized by the retinoscopist. This is akin to the principle that the meridian of power in a cylindrical lens is 90 degrees away from its axis.

Working Distance

The distance from the retinoscope to the patient's eye is known as the working distance. It is an important component to consider when performing retinoscopy. This is the distance at which the eye is focused when the reflex has been neutralized. It would be nice if this were equal to the standard distance for measuring visual acuity (20 feet or 6 m). However, it is virtually impossible to perform retinoscopy from that distance. The reflex appears very small, and it is difficult

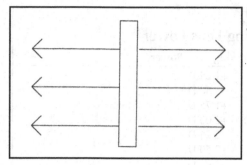

Figure 2-6. Retinoscope intercept oriented vertically and swept horizontally.

and time-consuming to change lenses. Therefore, retinoscopy is generally performed at an arm's length from the refractor.

The length of the average person's arm is 66 cm. The power of a lens that focuses parallel light rays at 66 cm is +1.50 D (you remember that D = 1 ÷ F, right?). In other words, the eye on which you just performed retinoscopy has 1.50 D of plus-powered *sphere* more than it needs (unless you want to measure visual acuity at 66 cm). To allow the eye to focus at 20 feet (6 m), this power must be taken away from the gross retinoscopy result. This is done by dialing 1.50 D toward the minus, also known as "removing the working lens." Some retinoscopists prefer to use the "retinoscopy lens" built into most refractors; the lens is inserted prior to performing retinoscopy and simply removed at the completion. There are two disadvantages to using the retinoscopy lens: it creates an additional reflex to dodge around, and it is a constant power (usually 1.50 D), making it less convenient for people with short arms or for radical retinoscopy (discussed later).

Some retinoscopists do not have arms that are 66 cm long. If your arms are shorter, say 57 cm, you will need to use a working lens of 1.75 D. That is, you need to remove 1.75 D of plus-powered *sphere* when you are done performing retinoscopy. People with really long arms (80 cm) will use a working lens of 1.25 D. If you are uncertain what your working distance is, you can extend a piece of string from the refractor to your eye while pretending to perform retinoscopy. Then, keeping your fingers on the string to mark the two points (denoting where the refractor and your eye were), stretch the string across a measuring stick. If the distance is between 54 and 61 cm, use 1.75 D as your working lens. Those with a working distance between 62 and 72 cm should use 1.50 D. Alternately, you may use a working lens as noted in Table 2-1.

It is imperative that you maintain this working distance while neutralizing the reflex. Changing the distance will cause you to change the power of your working lens. Yet, it may be necessary to alter your working distance at times, especially when working on eyes with very small pupils or opacities in the optical media. Just remember to change the power of your working lens accordingly.

What the Patient Needs to Know

- The retinoscope helps determine your glasses prescription.
- Just keep both eyes open and look at the letters on the chart, even if they are blurry.
- Do not look at the light.
- You can blink whenever you need to.
- Let me know if I block your view of the letters.

Table 2-1.
Determining Working Lens Power

Distance to Retinoscope	Working Lens Power
80 cm (0.8 m)	+1.25 D
67 cm (0.67 m)	+1.50 D
57 cm (0.57 m)	+1.75 D
50 cm (0.5 m)	+2.00 D
44 cm (0.44 m)	+2.25 D
40 cm (0.4 m)	+2.50 D
33 cm (0.33 m)	+3.00 D
25 cm (0.25 m)	+4.00 D
20 cm (0.20 m)	+5.00 D
16 cm (0.16 m)	+6.00 D
10 cm (0.10 m)	+10.00 D

Reflex Movement

The concept of retinoscopy is based on movement of the reflex. The objective is to find the lens(es) that will stop that movement. The two principal options for movement are "with" and "against." The retinoscopist must remember which lens (plus or minus) neutralizes each type of movement. This can be done by sheer memorization or by understanding how the reflex is formed.

The light from the retinoscope is shone into the eye and reflected by the retina. The image of this reflection, known as the reflex, will move either in the same direction as the intercept (with-movement) or in the opposite direction (against-movement). The direction of movement is dependent on where the focal point of the image is in relation to the retinoscope (Figure 2-7). If the focal point falls between the eye being examined and the retinoscope, the light rays will cross, the image will become inverted at the retinoscope, and against-movement is seen. With-movement is seen if the focal point is beyond the retinoscope; since the light has not come to a focal point, the rays have not crossed and, therefore, are not inverted. No movement of the reflex is seen if the focal point is *at* the retinoscope.

Now for the statement that you can memorize about the direction of movement. If you see with-movement, add plus-powered lenses. Conversely, against-movement is neutralized with minus-powered lenses. In certain cases, the movement of the reflex may appear to be skewed from that of the intercept (Figure 2-8). This is an indication that astigmatism is present, and the axis of the primary meridian is not parallel to the axis of the intercept. This will be discussed further in the "Procedure" section.

In addition to the direction of movement, the retinoscopist should assess the speed and brightness of the reflex. A dull, slow-moving reflex is seen when there is a significant refractive error. (In fact, a high refractive error may look neutral.) When neutrality is approached, the reflex quickens and becomes brighter. These are useful clues to grossly estimate the amount of refractive error and can lessen the amount of time required to perform retinoscopy. For example, when the retinoscopist sees against-movement, but it is dim and slow-moving, it can be postulated that a significant amount of myopia is present. An experienced retinoscopist would then place a high minus-powered lens in front of the patient's eye (rather than using small increments) and reassess the reflex.

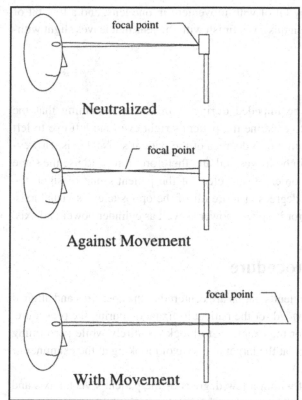

focal point

Neutralized

focal point

Against Movement

focal point

With Movement

Figure 2-7. Position of focal point in relation to direction of movement of the reflex.

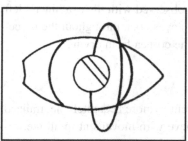

Figure 2-8. Misaligned streak. (Drawing by Holly Hess. Reprinted with permission from Ledford J. *Exercises in Refractometry.* Thorofare, NJ: SLACK Incorporated; 1990.)

Scissors Movement

Scissors movement is a reflex that seems to split and move in opposite directions. This type of movement is often seen in eyes with distorted corneas or large pupils. It can also be seen in eyes with a moderate to high amount of astigmatism where the axis is not parallel to the intercept. When scissors movement is seen, the intercept should be rotated in an attempt to align it with one of the primary meridians. If this fails to eliminate the confusing movement, the retinoscopist must concentrate on the central reflex.

Neutrality

The whole objective of retinoscopy is to achieve neutrality—that point where the reflex appears to have no movement. When the intercept enters the pupil, the reflex fills the pupil. The reflex then disappears when the intercept exits the pupil. Many times, true neutrality will not be achieved. Instead, there appears to be a tiny bit of with-movement in one lens, and a tiny bit of against-movement when +0.25 D is added. In this case, finish with the lens that leaves slight with-movement.

Visual Axis

The patient's visual axis should not be impeded during retinoscopy. Assuming that the retinoscopist is using his or her right eye to examine the patient's right eye (and left eye to left eye), it is easy to perform retinoscopy within 2 or 3 degrees of the patient's visual axis. However, not all retinoscopists have good vision in both eyes and are, therefore, forced to use the same eye to perform retinoscopy bilaterally. In order to stay clear of the patient's line of sight, the monocular retinoscopist is obliged to be 5 degrees or more off of the opposite eye's visual axis. This should be recognized as a source of error in sphere power as well as cylinder power and axis.

Procedure

The refractor is positioned so that the patient's pupils are centered in the apertures and aligned with the visual acuity chart. A target is provided for the patient to fixate on during the procedure. The larger the target, the less likely it is for the examiner to block it entirely while performing retinoscopy. The patient is instructed to look at the target and to avoid looking at the examiner or the retinoscope (to prevent accommodation).

The examiner positions him- or herself within a few degrees of the patient's visual axis and an arm's length away. As discussed earlier, the retinoscopist's right eye is used to examine the patient's right eye, and the reflex from the patient's left eye is observed with the examiner's left eye. It is recommended that the examiner and patient keep both eyes open throughout the procedure. The patient should be told to blink periodically to keep the cornea from drying.

Spherical Ametropia

Since it is agreed by most retinoscopists that with-movement is more accurately neutralized than against-movement, the first step in retinoscopy is to achieve with-movement in all meridians. When against-movement is seen at the start of retinoscopy, minus-powered sphere is added until with-movement is seen. Then plus-powered sphere is added until the reflex is neutralized. When there is no astigmatism present, the reflex will be neutralized at any axis.

Astigmatism

There are not too many eyes that have absolutely no astigmatism. Granted, some eyes have only 0.25 D of astigmatism, but they still have it. In fact, retinoscopy can *save time* during subjective refinement in eyes with very low amounts of astigmatism. Subjectively locating the axis with minimal cylinder power can be a time-consuming and sometimes confusing task for the patient during refractometry.

The majority of eyes have with-the-rule astigmatism (plus cylinder axis close to 90 degrees, or minus cylinder axis close to 180 degrees). Therefore, it is probably best to first assess the vertical meridian when using plus cylinder, or the horizontal meridian in the case of minus cylinder refractors. (More detail on neutralizing astigmatism is found in the following sections.)

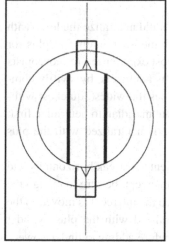

Figure 2-9. Correct alignment. Intercept, reflex, and cylinder axis are aligned.

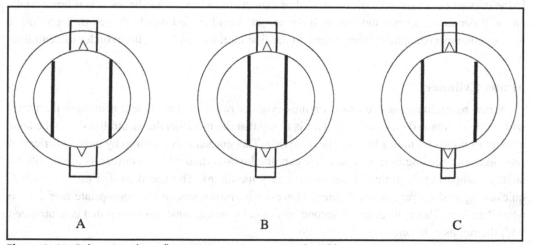

A   B   C

Figure 2-10. Enhancing the reflex. (A) Intercept at normal width. (B) Intercept is narrowed until the reflex is maximally narrowed. (C) Intercept has been narrowed too much, and reflex has become wider.

Astigmatism is recognized as a source of confusion for beginning retinoscopists. Try to think of the astigmatic eye as two separate eyes. One "eye" is neutralized with spherical lenses and the other "eye" with cylindrical lenses. The important thing to remember when neutralizing a reflex with cylindrical lenses is that the axis of the intercept, reflex, and cylinder must be parallel (Figure 2-9). The refractive error will not be properly neutralized if any one of the three components is not aligned.

Locating the exact axis of a primary meridian can be difficult when there is nominal astigmatism present. Enhancing (narrowing) the intercept can be of some assistance (Figure 2-10). For Copeland-style retinoscopes, lower the sleeve slightly until the intercept is *enhanced*. This narrowing of the intercept (and subsequently, the reflex) will make it easier to see the axis of the astigmatism. If the sleeve is lowered too far, the intercept will begin to widen again. For other styles of retinoscopes, raise the sleeve slightly.

Read the following section that pertains to your type of cylinder (plus or minus).

Plus Cylinder

When neutralizing an eye using a plus-cylinder refractor, one should neutralize the least-with (or most-against) meridian first. The meridian that neutralizes with the least amount of plus (or the most minus) is to be done first. This guideline is followed by most experienced retinoscopists because in most cases, they can quickly ascertain which meridian is applicable by swiftly comparing the reflex of the two primary meridians. The meridian that has the widest, quickest with-movement (or thinnest, slowest against-movement) is the appropriate meridian to neutralize first. This will set up the second meridian to have with-movement that is neutralized with the plus cylinder.

If this seems too confusing in the beginning, one may simply orient the streak horizontally and neutralize whatever is seen there. (If the reflex is off-axis from the intercept, be sure to realign the intercept before proceeding.) Then, in the majority of cases and when the intercept is moved to the vertical position, with-movement will be found and can be neutralized with the plus cylinder (remember to have the cylinder axis, intercept, and reflex aligned before adding cylinder power). In the minority of cases with against-the-rule astigmatism (where plus cylinder axis is horizontal), one will encounter against-movement in the second meridian and will be forced to neutralize it with minus-powered sphere. Then, return to the first meridian and use plus cylinder to neutralize it.

Minus Cylinder

When neutralizing an eye using a minus-cylinder refractor, one should neutralize the most-with (or least-against) meridian first. This is to say that the meridian that neutralizes with the least amount of minus (or most plus) is to be done first. This guideline is followed by most experienced retinoscopists because in most cases they can quickly ascertain which meridian is applicable by swiftly comparing the reflex of the two primary meridians. The meridian that has the widest, quickest against-movement (or thinnest, slowest with-movement) is the appropriate meridian to neutralize first. This will set up the second meridian to have against-movement that is neutralized with the minus cylinder.

If this seems too confusing in the beginning, one may simply orient the streak vertically and neutralize whatever is seen there. (If the reflex is off axis from your intercept, be sure to realign the intercept before proceeding.) Then, in the majority of cases and when the intercept is moved to the horizontal position, against-movement will be found and can be neutralized with the minus cylinder (remember to have the cylinder axis, intercept, and reflex aligned before adding cylinder power). Most retinoscopists prefer to add too much minus cylinder in order to achieve with-movement, then reduce the cylinder power until neutrality is obtained. In the minority of cases with against-the-rule astigmatism (where minus cylinder axis is vertical), one will encounter with-movement in the second meridian and will be forced to neutralize it with plus-powered sphere. Then, return to the first meridian and use minus cylinder to neutralize it.

Reversing Sleeve Position

There are a couple of reasons for reversing the position of the sleeve (all the way down for the Copeland retinoscopes or all the way up on the others). Some retinoscopists use this to verify neutrality (discussed next) while others use it to switch the movement of the reflex: against-movement becomes with-movement and vice versa. By reversing the movement, it is no longer necessary to add too much minus to produce with-movement. However, one must remember that the movement is not the only thing that has been reversed; the lens used to neutralize the reflex is also reversed (minus is used to neutralize with-movement, and plus is used to neutralize against-movement).

Verifying Neutrality

There are times when the reflex appears neutral, but in actuality, there is still a refractive error present. For example, when a high refractive error is present, the reflex may be moving so slowly that it appears to be neutralized; however, the reflex will also appear quite dim in this case. At other times, neutrality has almost been achieved but requires slightly more or less lens power for the reflex to be completely neutralized.

When a retinoscopist sees what he or she believes is a neutral reflex, it can be confirmed by reversing the sleeve position, adding extra lens power, or moving in and out from the usual working distance.

Reversing the sleeve position normally changes the direction of the reflex movement. If movement of the reflex is noted after reversing the sleeve position, then the reflex has not been neutralized. However, if the reflex has been neutralized, it will be neutral regardless of the sleeve position.

Adding additional lens power should cause movement of the reflex if it was previously neutralized. Although neutrality is often maintained over a small range (0.25 D), changing the lens power by 0.50 D should cause some movement of the reflex. If not, pseudo-neutrality may have been achieved, and a large refractive error still remains to be neutralized.

Moving in and out from the initial working distance is very similar to changing the lens power. Moving in slightly should result in with-movement; moving back beyond the working distance should cause against-movement. If this occurs, neutrality has been achieved. Otherwise, further work needs to be done.

Radical Retinoscopy

When performing retinoscopy on eyes that have small pupils or opaque media, seeing a reflex at the normal working distance can be difficult or impossible. Decreasing the working distance may allow the retinoscopist to see a reflex that can be neutralized from the new working distance.

Two potential sources of error are exacerbated by radical retinoscopy:

- It is easy to stray from the patient's visual axis by several degrees, inducing rather large errors. By constantly comparing his or her line of sight with the patient's visual axis, the retinoscopist should be able to avoid straying too far off axis.
- It is more difficult to determine the power of the working lens when using short distances. That is, when assuming a working distance of 66 cm, if the retinoscopist is actually using a distance of 63 cm, the change results in only a 0.07 D error. However, during radical retinoscopy, if the retinoscopist estimates the working distance to be 12 cm, but it is actually 9 cm, a 2.78 D error results. Unless he or she is very good at estimating small distances, the retinoscopist may need to use a ruler or other measuring device to ensure accurate measurement.

Upon completion of radical retinoscopy, the working lens is removed in the traditional manner. The only difference is in the power of the working lens. The power of the working lens, as mentioned before, is determined by using the formula $D = 1 \div F$. A working distance of 20 cm is equal to 5.00 D for the working lens, 15 cm is 6.67 D, and 10 cm is 10.00 D.

Figure 2-11. Fixation target for dynamic retinoscopy. (Photo courtesy of Welch Allyn, Inc.)

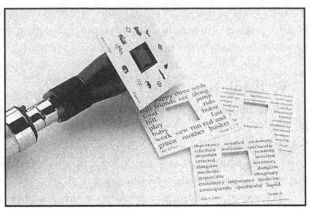

Dynamic Retinoscopy

Dynamic retinoscopy determines the refractive error at the distance of the retinoscope and essentially eliminates the working distance lens. First, retinoscopy is performed as usual with the patient looking in the distance. This measurement is called the static retinoscopy finding. Then, the patient is instructed to fixate on a target on the retinoscope (or in the same plane as the retinoscope), and the reflex is neutralized in the usual fashion (Figure 2-11). The amount of plus sphere power that is added beyond the static retinoscopy finding is the patient's lag of accommodation. This is a clue that the patient may need reading glasses or bifocals.

There are numerous methods of dynamic retinoscopy. Some methods stipulate that plus lenses are added until reversal of the reflex (from with-movement to against-movement) is achieved. One method (Sheard's) suggests that there is a normal lag of 0.50 D, and this amount should be subtracted from the dynamic retinoscopy findings. For example, if static retinoscopy showed -3.00 and the dynamic retinoscopy was -1.00, a +2.00 addition would be required for reading. According to Sheard, 0.50 would be subtracted, leaving an add of +1.50. Other methods indicate that the lag of accommodation is higher (up to 1.00 D).

New retinoscopes are often packaged with dynamic retinoscopy cards. These cards have various fixation targets surrounding a hole in the middle. The card is attached to the retinoscope so that the light shines through the hole.

Refining Cylinder Axis and Power

Using the retinoscope to refine the cylinder axis and power can save time during the subjective refinement process. With practice, refining the cylinder can be done in seconds. During the objective refinement, the retinoscopist shortens the working distance adequately to see with-movement in a previously neutralized eye.

Cylinder Axis—Straddle Cross Method

Position the intercept 45 degrees away from the cylinder axis. With-movement should still be seen. (If not, shorten the working distance further.) Note the width of the reflex at this axis. Now rotate the intercept 90 degrees so it is located 45 degrees to the other side of the cylinder axis.

What you have done is straddled the axis 45 degrees to either side.) Compare the width of the reflex at this axis to the previous reflex. If a difference is present, there is an error in the location of the cylinder axis. For plus cylinder units, rotate the cylinder axis toward the axis where the intercept was thinnest. Conversely, minus cylinder units should have the cylinder axis rotated toward the axis where the intercept was widest.

Repeat these steps until the reflex is of equal width 45 degrees on either side of the cylinder axis. Ensure that the intercept is positioned properly. The most common error with this technique is to inaccurately position the intercept.

Cylinder Power

Maintain the working distance used in the straddling technique. Rotate the intercept so that it is parallel to the cylinder axis. Note the width of the reflex. Next, rotate the intercept so that it is perpendicular to the cylinder axis. Compare the width of this reflex to the previous reflex. An error in cylinder power will be demonstrated by an inequality of the reflex width in each position.

If the width of the reflex parallel to the cylinder axis is narrower, the plus cylinder power must be increased or the minus cylinder power decreased. It may help to recall that increasing plus-power *decreases* with-movement (making the reflex wider). As expected, if the width of the reflex parallel to the cylinder axis is wider, the plus cylinder power needs to be decreased or the minus cylinder power increased.

Repeat these steps until the reflex parallel to the cylinder axis matches the width of the reflex perpendicular to the cylinder axis. If any changes were made to the cylinder power, the sphere power should be reconfirmed by returning to the normal working distance and neutralizing the reflex, if necessary.

Estimation Technique

Under normal circumstances, retinoscopy is performed on cooperative patients, and a refractor is used for lens selection. However, if loose lenses are used or the patient has a very short attention span, it is helpful to be able to estimate the refractive error before lenses are introduced. Jack Copeland had exceptional skill in this area, but not many other retinoscopists have mastered the estimation technique (also known as spiraling). The availability of refractors has drastically reduced the demand for learning the estimation technique.

Using two hands is permitted, and even recommended, while spiraling. The intercept is rotated each time the sleeve is moved vertically by 0.5 mm. This allows the retinoscopist to determine if astigmatism is present and, if so, where the principal meridians are located.

Myopia

Less Than 5.00 Diopters

This category is the easiest to estimate since it is done merely by determining the distance between the eye and retinoscope that neutralization occurs. The patient is asked to fixate on a distant target while the retinoscopist varies the working distance until the reflex is neutral. Using the formula $D = 1 \div F$, the amount of myopia is determined. For example, if the reflex neutralizes with the retinoscope held 33 cm from the eye, the amount of myopia is 3.00 D ($D = 1 \div 0.33$) (Table 2-2).

Table 2-2.
Estimating Myopia Without Lenses

Eye to Retinoscope Distance	Amount of Myopia
10 cm (0.1 m)	10.00 D
12.5 cm (0.125 m)	8.00 D
16 cm (0.16 m)	6.00 D
20 cm (0.2 m)	5.00 D
25 cm (0.25 m)	4.00 D
33 cm (0.33 m)	3.00 D
40 cm (0.4 m)	2.50 D
44 cm (0.44 m)	2.25 D
50 cm (0.5 m)	2.00 D
57 cm (0.57m)	1.75 D
67 cm (0.67 m)	1.50 D
80 cm (0.8 m)	1.25 D

Figure 2-12. Estimating myopia >5.00 D.

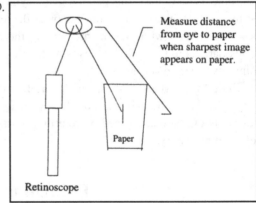

Measure distance from eye to paper when sharpest image appears on paper.

Paper

Retinoscope

More Than 5.00 Diopters

The reflex is dim and difficult to see when the eye has more than 5.00 D of myopia. The reflex can be brightened by reversing the sleeve position to create a concave-mirror effect. This also reverses the direction of movement of the reflex. The retinoscopist moves inward toward the patient until the reflex is enhanced (narrowed). When the best quality of the reflex is seen, a piece of white paper is positioned adjacent to the light source of the retinoscope, and an image of the bulb filament (reflected from the eye) is seen (Figure 2-12). The distance that the paper is held from the eye to achieve the sharpest image is used to convert to D (see previous heading on p. 43 "Less Than 5.00 Diopters").

Exercises

For the following exercises, you will need a retinoscope, schematic eye, and a trial lens set with plus and minus cylinders. (If your trial lens set does not have both plus and minus cylinders, see "Special Notes" at the end of this section.) A refractor would be beneficial, but it is not critical that you have one. If a refractor is available to you, tape the schematic eye to the headrest of the exam chair and place the refractor as close to the lens holder of the schematic eye as possible for Exercises 2 through 8.

Exercise 1

Position the schematic eye an arm's length away from you. Using the retinoscope with the sleeve in the proper position, and neutralize the schematic eye by making it longer or shorter. If with-movement is seen, the eye is hyperopic (too short) in relation to your working distance, and must be lengthened. Conversely, against-movement signifies myopia (schematic eye is too long) and the eye should be shortened until neutralization results.

Assuming you have a working distance close to 66 cm and the markings on the schematic eye are accurate, -1.50 (or 1.50 D of myopia) should be showing on the scale. However, be aware that the scale for schematic eyes is not famous for its accuracy. So, rather than rely on a scale to prove that you are neutral, use the techniques described in this chapter. Try reversing the sleeve position. Also try moving in and out slightly from your normal working distance. Now is the time to become familiar with these verification techniques.

Exercise 2

Leaving the eye neutralized from Exercise 1, place a -2.00 sphere in the lens holder of the schematic eye. This should produce some obvious with-movement. Neutralize this movement with the appropriately powered sphere, using 0.50 D increments to demonstrate the characteristics of the reflex as neutrality is approached. The first 1.00 D will likely have nominal effect on the appearance of the reflex. The next 0.50 D will show how the reflex widens and the movement becomes faster. The final 0.50 D (for a total of +2.00 D) should neutralize the reflex.

Exercise 3

Remove the lenses used in Exercise 2, but maintain the length of the schematic eye. Now, place a +3.00 D spherical trial lens into the holder of the schematic eye. Assume your normal working distance, and sweep the intercept across the pupil. It may be necessary to move the intercept fluently from side-to-side, exiting the pupil on each side, to find the expected against-movement. Otherwise, some schematic eyes may appear as though they are neutral. Do at least one of the verification techniques to determine that the eye is not truly neutralized.

Just as you did in Exercise 2, use 0.50 D increments (of the opposite power, naturally) until the eye is neutralized. If you agree with the majority of retinoscopists that against-movement is more difficult to neutralize than with-movement, add an extra 0.50 D to obtain with-movement, then reduce the power using 0.25 D increments until neutrality occurs.

Exercise 4

Remove the trial lens(es) used in the previous exercise and place a +10.00 trial lens in the lens holder. The reflex will now take on a dimmer appearance. It may also appear as though there is with-movement; this is an artifact seen on schematic eyes due to their simple optics (you are only seeing the edge of the intercept, and it will be continuous with the edge of the reflex). If this is the case, reverse the sleeve position and a brighter, thinner, with-movement will be seen, proving that the original reflex did not truly have with-movement. Return the sleeve to the proper position. You could also try drastically shortening your working distance (to about 15 cm) and note against-movement.

Add minus-powered sphere until with-movement is seen. Then reduce the power in 0.25 D increments until neutrality occurs (this can be done by using the plus low-powered spheres placed in front of the minus-sphere lens). If you are using trial lenses to neutralize the reflex, use 1.00 D increments and begin at -5.00. Due to the vertex distance, the powers may not match exactly. It is not unusual to require -10.50 (or even more) to neutralize the refractive error created by the +10.00 trial lens.

Exercise 5

Remove all lenses. After ensuring that the schematic eye is still neutralized, insert a -10.00 sphere. This will simulate an eye with high hyperopia. Due to the simple optics of the schematic eye, you will likely see a reflex very similar to that which was seen at the beginning of Exercise 4 (dim, with-movement). Reversing the sleeve in this scenario will produce a thinner reflex, but it will still be the exact same width as the intercept. In a human eye, the movement of the reflex would have been reversed to create against-movement.

Begin adding plus-powered sphere until the reflex is neutralized. If you are using trial lenses to neutralize, use 1.00 D increments and begin at +5.00. When the reflex appears neutralized, use one of the verification techniques to ensure that the reflex is truly neutralized.

Exercise 6

Remove the trial lens(es) used in Exercise 5, and place a -1.25 cylinder with its axis at 90 degrees. (Do not change the length of the eye.) With the intercept positioned horizontally, the eye should still appear neutralized. Rotate the intercept to the vertical position (parallel to the cylinder axis) and with-movement should be seen. This is simple hyperopic, with-the-rule astigmatism and is neutralized with a plus cylinder at 90 degrees. (If you are using a minus cylinder refractor, you will first have to add +1.25 sphere, then use minus cylinder at 180 degrees.)

Remove all lenses except the -1.25 cylinder. Rotate the cylinder axis to 80 degrees. Position your intercept at 90 degrees, and sweep across the aperture. The reflex should appear tilted clockwise to the position of the intercept. When the intercept and reflex are not parallel, the intercept should be rotated until it is aligned with the reflex. This will also make the reflex brighter and sharper. Then, before adding cylinder power, position the correcting cylinder axis to match that of the intercept. Practice by neutralizing the schematic eye now.

Exercise 7

Remove the trial lens(es) from the lens holder of the schematic eye. Lengthen the eye slightly and use the retinoscope to ensure that against-movement is seen. Now place 2.00 D of minus cylinder in the lens holder with the axis at 120. With the intercept in the horizontal position (180 degrees), sweep across the aperture. The reflex may be a bit confusing and may not follow the direction of your intercept because you are not aligned with one of the primary meridians. Slowly rotate the intercept 360 degrees while sweeping across the aperture. This allows you to quickly survey the situation; you should find the best quality with-movement at 120 degrees (if this is not the case, the eye was lengthened too much and should be shortened somewhat). The best quality against-movement will be seen at 30 degrees. Choose the appropriate meridian and neutralize it with spheres. If you are using plus cylinder, you should position your intercept at 30 degrees. Those using minus cylinder refractors should position their intercept at 120 degrees.

Now, "half" of the eye has been neutralized. All that remains is astigmatism. Rotate the intercept 90 degrees and use cylindrical lenses to neutralize. You are done!

Obviously, the human eye does not have markings on it to show the axis of the astigmatism. It is beneficial to refine the cylinder axis and power with the retinoscope, as described earlier in this chapter.

Exercise 8

Remove all the trial lenses and shorten the schematic eye sufficiently to obtain some with-movement. Then, place a -2.00 cylinder into the lens holder, and position the axis at 170 degrees. This simulates compound hyperopic astigmatism. All meridians should display with-movement.

For those using plus-cylinder refractors, attempt to locate the axis with the least-with (widest reflex). Those using minus-cylinder refractors should locate the most-with axis first. Use spherical lenses to neutralize this axis. For greatest accuracy, ensure your reflex and intercept are parallel.

Rotate the intercept 90 degrees. Now you should see the appropriate movement (with-movement for plus cylinder refractors or against-movement for minus cylinder). Neutralize this using cylindrical lenses while keeping the axis of the intercept, reflex, and cylinder parallel.

Exercise 9

Create your own situations with the schematic eye, and neutralize them. If possible, have an experienced retinoscopist verify your findings.

Special Notes

What to Do if Only Plus Cylinder is Available

Some ophthalmology/optometry offices use a trial lens set that has only plus cylinders. In this case, a modification must be made to the exercises. Place the cylinder axis 90 degrees from the axis indicated. For example, if you are using a plus cylinder refractor and have only plus cylinder trial lenses, the trial lens cylinder will be positioned with its axis perpendicular to the intended axis. That is, if the exercise indicates an axis of 90 degrees, the trial lens should be at 180 degrees. This will allow you to follow the exercise and use the correcting cylinder at the proper axis. (In this case, the correcting cylinder would still be placed at axis 90 degrees.)

In addition to changing the axis, the sphere power should also be altered by the same amount as the cylinder power. For example, Exercise 7 asks you to place a -2.00 cylinder at 120 degrees; you will instead use a plus cylinder of the same power at 30 degrees. By adding a +2.00 cylinder, the sphere should be increased by -2.00 (simply select a sphere that has the same power but opposite sign as the cylinder).

Chapter 3

Refractometry

- Refractometry refinement should be done in the following order—cylinder axis, cylinder power, and sphere power.

- The cylinder axis of two eyes (that have not had any surgery) usually adds up to 180. (Eg, if the cylinder axis of one eye is 40, the cylinder axis of the fellow eye will often be close to 140.)

- For best results, the patient should understand what the examiner is trying to achieve during refractometry and how he or she is expected to respond.

- The cross cylinder usually causes the patient's vision to be slightly blurred; he or she should be made aware that this is normal and choose which is sharper of the next two choices.

- "Push plus" means to use the maximum amount of plus-powered sphere (or minimum minus-powered sphere) to achieve best acuity.

Introduction

Refractometry is the measurement of the refractive error of an eye. Technicians are often utilized for this task. Computers (automated refractometers) can objectively measure the refractive error. Licensed professionals, such as an optometrist or ophthalmologist, can do *refractions*. The difference between refractometry and refraction is in the final decision-making process. There are times when the lenses that provide the sharpest vision are not the same lenses that will create the best spectacles. For example, there may be a significant anisometropia (different refractive error in each eye) that may cause aniseikonia (different sized image in each eye). This would not likely be tolerated by the patient. It is up to the licensed professional to decide which lenses will provide the best result under the given circumstances. A technician who does refractions is practicing medicine without a license.

The basic steps of refractometry can be described in a single sentence. First, estimate the spherical component, then refine the cylinder axis and power, and finally, refine the sphere power. Unfortunately, it is not that easy to teach or learn. This chapter describes the steps in detail using plus and minus cylinder techniques. Practice the process on fellow staff, friends, relatives—whoever is willing to sit still for a while. This is preferable to using patients, until your confidence is established.

Anatomy of the Refractor

The refractor (or phoropter) is an instrument that houses various lenses that can be used to determine the refractive error of an eye, as well as for some orthoptic tests. Prior to the invention of the refractor, examiners were required to use loose lenses—a tedious task for most people.

Before one performs refractometry, it is necessary to know the controls on the refractor (Figure 3-1). Not all refractors are the same, but they all have the essential features (controls to adjust sphere, cylinder axis, cylinder power, and an occluder). Some, like the instrument shown in Figure 3-1, have auxiliary lenses to increase efficiency. Consult the operator's manual for your specific model.

Preparing the Patient

Take a minute or two to explain the procedure to the patient. Let him or her know what will be done, why it will be done, and what to expect as a response. After giving this speech a few hundred times, it may become monotonous. Regardless, it will usually save a lot of grief during the refractometry process.

There is not a single description that works for every patient. Some personalities want to know absolutely everything about what you are going to do. It may seem that they could quite possibly perform the test themselves by the time you are done. Others want the bare necessities; after all, time is money. However, there are key points you want to discuss in almost every case; these are presented in "What the Patient Needs to Know" on p51.

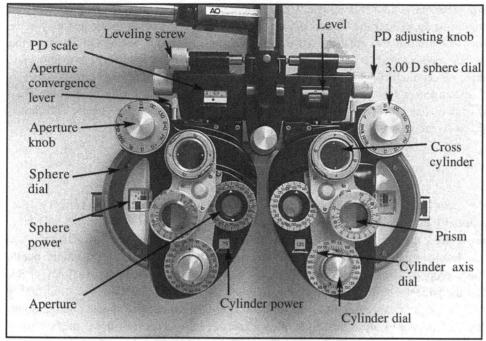

Figure 3-1. Refractor front (labeled). (Reprinted with permission from Ledford J. *Exercises in Refractometry.* Thorofare, NJ: SLACK Incorporated; 1990.)

What the Patient Needs to Know

- The procedure is used to select the lens that provides the clearest vision.

- For each choice, please indicate which is clearer.

- Sometimes the choices may look the same. In that case, just say that you cannot tell the difference.

- Do not worry about making a mistake. The examiner tests a lens more than once.

- If the lenses move too quickly, ask the examiner to slow down.

- If you do not understand what you are being asked, tell the examiner.

Which One Is Better?

The question always arises, what do I label each lens choice? Do I always say, "Which one is better—one, or two?" Or should I increase the number each time, "Now, which one is better—three, or four?" There is no correct response to this question. It is mostly a matter of personal preference, with some variation for special cases.

There is a risk that some patients who, despite a good explanation at the beginning of the test, will select the same choice each time. For example, if the patient's first selection is "number one," each subsequent choice may also be "number one." If you prefer to be consistent with numbering the lenses, you may still find occasions when you need to either alter the numbers or "trick" the patient by reversing the choices—switch the order of presentation of the lenses so that the lens that was number one is now number two. If the patient has been constantly picking number one and continues to do so after the choices are reversed, a better explanation of the test may be in order. This scenario can also present itself if the patient has difficulties seeing the letters on the eye chart; both choices are blurry and the patient is only guessing. Ask the patient to read the letters again to be certain they are legible.

Some examiners prefer to alternate between letters and numbers to avoid any confusion. They use "one or two" one time, then "a or b" the next, and return to "one or two" again. The choice is yours. Use whatever works best for you and the patient.

Aligning the Refractor

The refractor has a few controls that allow it to be aligned properly with the patient's eyes. The unit usually extends from a pivot arm that allows gross alignment with the patient's face. Then the pupillary distance is adjusted so each eye is centered within the aperture. The refractor can also be leveled using the built-in level as a guide. When the instrument is level and the pupillary distance properly set, each eye should look through the center of the aperture. If not, check to see that the patient's head is not tilted. Please note that some patients have one orbit that is higher than the other. In this case, tilting the refractor is *not* the appropriate way to align it. Some units allow the operator to adjust the height of each aperture independently—this is the best solution. However, if your unit does not have this feature, you will be forced to refract one eye, and then adjust the height of the refractor before completing the test on the fellow eye.

Finally, before beginning the test, occlude the eye that is not being tested. You may forget to do this once in a while and the patient will have difficulty discerning any changes in lenses since the fellow eye's vision will remain consistent. Be alert to this clue, and check to see that the fellow eye is occluded before becoming aggravated over what appears to be a patient's lack of attention to detail.

Starting Point

It is quite time-consuming to start refracting without an appropriate starting point. There are various methods to determine the starting point:

- Retinoscopy (discussed in Chapter 2).
- Autorefractor.
- Prescription of the patient's habitual spectacles (from lensometry).
- Refractometry results from a previous visit.
- Keratometry (to estimate cylinder component—best used for postoperative cataract surgery where the spherical equivalent is hopefully close to plane, and no lenticular astigmatism is expected).

Unless retinoscopy is to be used, it may be best to place the starting point in the refractor before positioning the unit in front of the patient. This will prevent unnecessary visual distortions because the lenses are changed from the previous patient's results to the current patient's refractive error. In the case of retinoscopy, it is advisable to begin without any lenses in place (except maybe the retinoscopy working lens).

Initial Determination of Sphere

OphT

Despite the examiner's best efforts to choose the appropriate starting point, it is still possible that the sphere and/or cylinder component are not correct. Before changing any lenses, determine what the patient is capable of seeing with the current lens selection. The patient should be asked to concentrate on a line that is somewhat difficult to read. Then the sphere is changed in appropriate increments: 0.25 D for vision that is 20/40 or better; 0.50 D for 20/50 to 20/100; and 1.00 D (or possibly more) for those with vision less than 20/100. The first change in sphere should be towards the plus—continue in the plus direction until vision begins to blur. If the first change in the plus direction caused blurring, return to the starting point, and then go in the minus direction. Continue in the minus direction until the next change provides no further improvement.

During refractometry, the examiner should always "push plus." This means to use the highest plus- (or least minus-) powered sphere lens that affords the best vision. It is not possible to use more plus than required. However, since accommodation can overcome minus-powered spheres, it is quite easy to "over minus." Assuming that the patient has relatively good vision in the eye being tested, each addition of minus-powered spheres should result in an improvement in the sharpness of the letters. This can be verified by asking the patient to read further down the eye chart as minus sphere is increased (or plus sphere is reduced). One tell-tale sign that the patient is beginning to use accommodation is that the letters appear smaller or darker, but not any sharper. Fogging (cyclodamia)—a procedure to ensure that maximum plus sphere has been used—will be discussed later in this chapter.

Cylinder Refinement

Since refractors are equipped with either plus or minus cylinders (but not both), it is easier if the two methods of correcting astigmatism are separated here. *Read only the appropriate section.* For those uncertain whether they are using plus or minus cylinders, look at the color of the numbers that indicate the cylinder power—black numbers are used for plus cylinder and red numbers for minus cylinder.

Plus Cylinder Technique

Before it is possible to accurately determine the cylinder power, the cylinder axis must be refined. (It does no good to try to refine cylinder power unless the axis is already correct.) There are two common methods used to help the patient choose the proper cylinder axis: the astigmatic dial and the cross cylinder technique. The latter is the most popular (and possibly the most accurate) method. The astigmatic dial is most commonly used to determine the gross axis and cylinder power, which may be further refined with the cross cylinder. Neither method should be considered appropriate for use with all patients.

OphT

The location of the cylinder axis becomes more critical with increasing amounts of astigmatism. For example, if the axis is moved 10 degrees with 0.50 D of cylinder in place, the vision will not change dramatically. However, moving the axis the same amount when the cylinder power is 5.00 D will significantly change the patient's vision. Therefore, more care must be taken when refining the cylinder axis in higher amounts of astigmatism. You can demonstrate this to yourself by using trial lenses of various cylinder powers and rotating each one as you look through it.

OphT

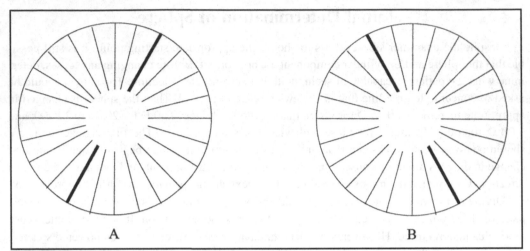

Figure 3-2. Astigmatic dial. When using a mirror system, the "clock hours" will be reversed.

 Astigmatic Dial

The astigmatic dial is a chart with radial lines. The patient is asked to report which, if any, lines appear blackest or sharpest. Ensure that no cylinder power is in place at the beginning of this procedure. It is also necessary to "fog" the patient by adding +0.50 D to the sphere that was estimated using the previous step. If all lines appear equal, add another +0.25 D sphere. If all lines still appear equal, introduce +0.50 cylinder at 90 degrees; the horizontal lines should then appear sharper, confirming that the patient is able to properly respond to this test and that no visually significant astigmatism is present.

If some lines do appear blacker or sharper (before adding any cylinder power), the patient is asked to indicate the position of those lines using "clock hours." For example, if the lines running vertical are the blackest, the patient will say the lines going from 12:00 to 6:00 are the blackest. Position the cylinder axis parallel to (ie, in line with) this axis and begin adding cylinder power until all lines are equal. Please note that, when a mirror system is used, the face of the "clock" is reversed for the examiner. That is, if the lines running from 1:00 to 7:00 are the sharpest, the examiner will position the cylinder axis at 120 degrees (equivalent to the 11:00 position) (Figure 3-2). Add -0.25 D sphere for every 0.50 cylinder added to maintain the SE and keep the circle of least confusion in front of the retina.

Paraboline Test

It is not possible to refine the cylinder axis within a few degrees using the astigmatic dial alone. Some projectors have a paraboline slide (Figure 3-3) that is linked to the astigmatic dial. This can increase the accuracy in choosing the cylinder axis and power. The gross axis is determined with the astigmatic dial (or other means such as retinoscopy). When using the astigmatic dial, there may be an arrow that can be rotated using the projector control panel. It is positioned 90 degrees away from the lines that the patient indicated were the blackest or sharpest. Then the paraboline slide (curved lines that converge toward each other) is introduced. When using other means to estimate the cylinder axis, the dotted line of the paraboline that runs between the two curved lines is positioned at the estimated axis. The patient is asked to report which of the curved lines appears sharper. The paraboline slide is rotated *in the direction of* the sharper line, until both lines appear equal.

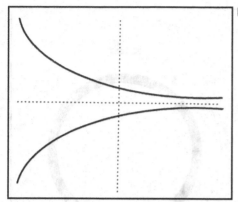

Figure 3-3. Paraboline chart.

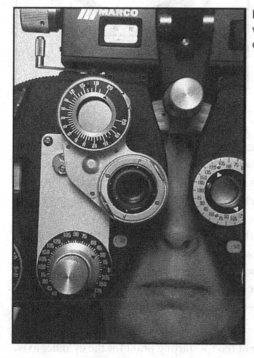

Figure 3-4. Cross cylinder. Knurled knob is aligned with correcting cylinder axis in preparation of refining cylinder axis.

Match the axis of the correcting cylinder to the axis of the paraboline slide. Begin to add cylinder power until the patient reports that both lines of the cross (consisting of dotted lines) appear equal. Remember to maintain the SE (adding -0.25 sphere for every 0.50 cylinder added). Remove the fogging lens power upon completion of this step.

Cross Cylinder Technique

OphT

The cross cylinder is a plus cylinder of a specific power (usually 0.25 D or 0.37 D) placed perpendicular to a minus cylinder of the same power. As mentioned earlier, the first step in refining the cylinder is to determine the correct axis. Using the cross cylinder, this is done by positioning its knurled knob (used to flip the lens) parallel with the correcting cylinder axis (Figure 3-4). This will place the axis of the plus cylinder in the cross cylinder 45 degrees to one side of the correcting cylinder axis, and the minus cylinder axis 45 degrees to the other side. When the lens is flipped, the position of the plus and minus cylinder axes trade places.

Figure 3-5. Refining cylinder axis. Correcting cylinder axis is rotated toward the white dot when cross cylinder displays patient's choice.

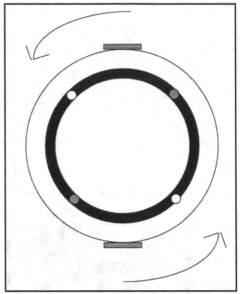

Ultimately, with each flip of the cross cylinder, the patient is able to see how the vision is affected as if the correcting cylinder is rotated in either direction. If the patient prefers one choice over the other, position the lens with the patient's favored choice showing by rotating the correcting cylinder axis several degrees in the direction of the white marker (Figure 3-5). This process is continued until the patient either reports no change when the lens is flipped, or repeatedly goes back and forth within a degree or two.

The patient should be advised that the vision will likely diminish somewhat with the introduction of the cross cylinder. This occurs because the axis of the cross cylinder is always to one side or the other of the correcting cylinder axis. Since the axis is never in alignment with the correcting cylinder and assuming that the axis of the correcting cylinder was reasonably close to being accurate, this will detract from the quality of vision by inducing some astigmatism.

Locating Approximate Axis

There will be occasions when the examiner will not have a starting point for the cylinder axis, or possibly be unaware whether astigmatism is present. The cross cylinder can be used to solve this problem. Without any cylinder power in place, the cross cylinder is positioned so that the red axis marker is at 90 degrees. (As usual, the patient is informed that his or her vision may be a bit worse.) Ask, "Of the next two choices, which seems sharper?" and flip the cross cylinder lens. If both are the same, then rotate the cross cylinder 45 degrees (now at 135 or 45 degrees) and again ask if one choice is better than the other. If the patient chooses one lens over the other, the correcting cylinder axis is positioned at the location of the white marker on the cross cylinder, and 0.50 D of cylinder is added (along with -0.25 sphere to maintain SE). Then the usual cross cylinder procedure (discussed previously) is used to refine the measurement. If none of the choices are any better than the rest, it can be assumed that there is not any visually significant astigmatism present. Please note that the visual acuity needs to be reasonably good (20/60 or better) for this procedure to work.

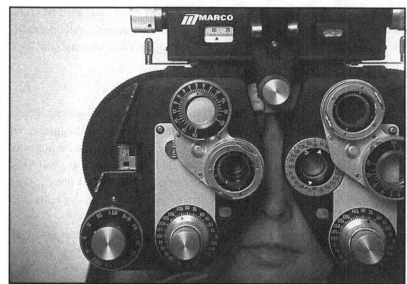

Figure 3-6. Cross cylinder. "P" on the cross cylinder is aligned with the correcting cylinder axis in preparation of refining cylinder power (when using a refractor that does not have "P" marking, align a white or red dot/line with the correcting cylinder axis).

Cylinder Power

Once the axis has been refined, it is time to fine-tune the cylinder power. The cross cylinder is rotated so that its axis is aligned with the correcting cylinder axis. Most refractors have a "P" (for power) on the rim of the cross cylinder for the purpose of alignment (Figure 3-6). Now, when the cross cylinder lens is flipped, the minus and plus cylinder axes will trade places (ie, either the minus or plus cylinder will be aligned with the correcting cylinder axis, depending on which side of the lens is being displayed).

If the vision is better when the white marker on the cross cylinder is aligned with the correcting cylinder, cylinder power should be increased. Conversely, the red marker indicates that the plus-cylinder power should be decreased. The process of adding or subtracting power is repeated until the patient indicates that both choices are equal or alternates between two choices repeatedly. In the latter case, the examiner may choose the cylinder power that the patient seems to prefer. For example, suppose the patient responds quickly when trying to decide if the cylinder power should be increased (eg, from 0.75 D to 1.00 D), but hesitates when the cross cylinder indicates that the cylinder power should be decreased (in this example, from 1.00 D back to 0.75 D). The choice would be 1.00 D. Otherwise, when in doubt, select the lower power.

Minus Cylinder Technique

Before it is possible to accurately determine the cylinder power, the cylinder axis must be refined. It does no good to try to refine cylinder power unless the axis is already correct. There are two common methods used to help the patient choose the proper cylinder axis—the astigmatic dial and the cross cylinder technique. The latter is the most popular (and possibly the most accurate) method, which may be further refined with the cross cylinder. The astigmatic dial is most commonly used to determine the gross axis and cylinder power. Neither method should be considered appropriate for use with all patients.

The location of the cylinder axis becomes more critical with increasing amounts of astigmatism. For example, if the axis is moved 10 degrees with 0.50 D of cylinder in place, the vision will not change dramatically. However, moving the axis the same amount when the cylinder

OphT

power is 5.00 D will significantly change the patient's vision. Therefore, more care must be taken when refining the cylinder axis in higher amounts of astigmatism. You can demonstrate this to yourself by using trial lenses of various cylinder powers and rotating each one as you look through it.

Astigmatic Dial

The astigmatic dial is a chart with radial lines. The patient is asked to report which, if any, lines appear blackest or sharpest. Ensure that no cylinder power is in place at the beginning of this procedure. It is also necessary to "fog" the patient by adding +0.50 D to the sphere that was estimated using the previous step. If all lines appear equal, add another +0.25 D sphere. If all lines still appear equal, introduce -0.50 cylinder at 90 degrees; the vertical lines should then appear sharper, confirming that the patient is able to properly respond to this test and that no visually significant astigmatism is present.

If some lines do appear blacker or sharper (before adding any cylinder power), the patient is asked to indicate the position of those lines using "clock hours." For example, if the lines running vertical are the blackest, the patient will say the lines going from 12:00 to 6:00 are the blackest. Position the cylinder axis perpendicular to (ie, 90 degrees from) this axis and begin adding cylinder power until all lines are equal. The "Rule of 30" may be used to calculate the axis: multiply the lower "clock hour" (in this example, 6:00) by 30; 6 x 30 = 180. Add +0.25 D sphere for every 0.50 cylinder added to maintain the SE and keep the circle of least confusion in front of the retina.

Paraboline Test

It is not possible to refine the cylinder axis within a few degrees using the astigmatic dial alone. Some projectors have a paraboline slide (see Figure 3-3) that is linked to the astigmatic dial. This can increase the accuracy in choosing the cylinder axis and power. The gross axis is determined with the astigmatic dial (or other means such as retinoscopy). When using the astigmatic dial, there may be an arrow that can be rotated using the projector control panel. It is used to point to the lines that the patient indicated were the blackest or sharpest. Then the paraboline slide (curved lines that converge toward each other) is introduced. When using other means to estimate the cylinder axis, the dotted line of the paraboline that runs between the two curved lines is positioned perpendicular to the estimated axis. The patient is asked to report which of the curved lines appears sharper. The paraboline slide is rotated *away* from the sharper line until both lines appear equal.

Position the axis of the correcting cylinder perpendicular to the axis of the paraboline slide. Then begin to add cylinder power until the patient reports that both lines of the cross (consisting of dotted lines) appear equal. Remember to maintain the SE (adding +0.25 sphere for every 0.50 cylinder added). Remove the fogging lens power upon completion of this step.

Cross Cylinder Technique

The Jackson cross cylinder is a minus cylinder of a specific power (usually 0.25 D or 0.37 D) placed perpendicular to a plus cylinder of the same power. As mentioned earlier, the first step in refining the cylinder is to determine the correct axis. Using the cross cylinder, this is done by positioning its knurled knob (used to flip the lens) parallel with the correcting cylinder axis (see Figure 3-4). This will place the axis of the minus cylinder in the cross cylinder 45 degrees to one side of the correcting cylinder axis, and the plus cylinder axis 45 degrees to the other side. When the lens is flipped, the position of the plus and minus cylinder axes trade places.

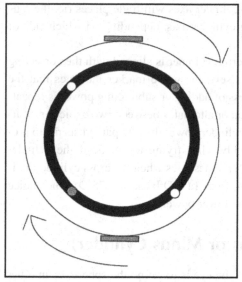

Figure 3-7. Refining cylinder axis. Correcting cylinder axis is rotated toward the red dot when cross cylinder displays patient's choice.

Ultimately, with each flip of the cross cylinder, the patient is able to see how the vision is affected as if the correcting cylinder is rotated in either direction. If the patient prefers one choice over the other, position the lens with the patient's favored choice showing. Rotate the correcting cylinder axis several degrees in the direction of the red marker (Figure 3-7). This process is repeated until the patient either reports no change when the lens is flipped or repeatedly goes back and forth within a degree or two.

The patient should be advised that the vision will likely diminish somewhat with the introduction of the cross cylinder. This occurs because the axis of the cross cylinder is always to one side or the other of the correcting cylinder axis. Since the axis is never in alignment with the correcting cylinder (and assuming the axis of the correcting cylinder was reasonably close to being accurate), this will detract from the quality of vision.

Locating Approximate Axis

There will be occasions when the examiner will not have a starting point for the cylinder axis or possibly be unaware whether or not astigmatism is present. The cross cylinder can also be used to solve this problem. Without any cylinder power in place, the cross cylinder is positioned so that the red axis marker is at 90 degrees. (As usual, the patient is informed that his or her vision may be a bit worse.) Ask, "Of the next two choices, which seems sharper?" and flip the cross cylinder lens. If both are the same, then rotate the cross cylinder 45 degrees (now at 135 or 45 degrees), and again ask if one choice is better than the other. If the patient chooses one lens over the other, the correcting cylinder axis is positioned at the location of the red marker on the cross cylinder, and 0.50 D of cylinder is added (along with +0.25 sphere to maintain SE). Then the usual cross cylinder procedure is used to refine the measurement. If none of the choices is any better than the rest, it can be assumed that there is not any visually significant astigmatism present. Please note that the visual acuity needs to be reasonably good (20/60 or better) for this procedure to work.

Cylinder Power

Once the axis has been refined, it is time to fine-tune the cylinder power. The cross cylinder is rotated so that its axis is aligned with the correcting cylinder axis. Most refractors have a "P" (for power) on the rim of the cross cylinder for purpose of alignment (see Figure 3-6). Now, when the cross cylinder lens is flipped, the plus and minus cylinder axes will trade places (ie, the plus or minus cylinder will be aligned with the correcting cylinder axis, depending on which side of the lens is being displayed).

If the vision is better when the red marker on the cross cylinder is aligned with the correcting cylinder, cylinder power should be increased. Conversely, the white marker indicates that the minus cylinder power should be decreased. The process of adding or subtracting power is repeated until the patient indicates that both choices are equal or alternates between two choices repeatedly. In the latter case, the examiner may choose the cylinder power that the patient seems to prefer. For example, suppose the patient responds quickly when trying to decide if the cylinder power should be increased (eg, from 0.75 D to 1.00 D) but hesitates when the cross cylinder indicates that the cylinder power should be decreased (eg, from 1.00 D back to 0.75 D). The choice would be 1.00 D. Otherwise, when in doubt, select the lower power.

Refining Sphere Power (Plus or Minus Cylinder)

The final step in measuring the refractive error of the eye is to refine the sphere, or in other words, determine the spherical end point. Remove the cross cylinder, display the acuity chart, and ask the patient to read the smallest line possible.

Now, fog the patient's vision by adding +1.00 sphere (or decrease the minus sphere by 1.00 D). Assuming that the patient was able to read 20/20 (or better) prior to fogging, the visual acuity should now be reduced to around 20/30 or 20/40. Ask the patient to concentrate on the lowest line that was read before the fog. As the fog is decreased (by adding minus sphere, 0.25 D at a time), instruct the patient to inform you when that line becomes legible (not necessarily clear). In the vision range of 20/40 to 20/15, each 0.25 D increment should improve vision by one line on the eye chart. It should only take an extra 0.25 D of minus sphere beyond the legible point to provide the best quality vision. Before adding that last 0.25 D, ask the patient to tell you whether the next lens makes the letters appear *sharper*, or just smaller or darker. Remember that accommodation causes letters to appear smaller and darker, and the idea is to prevent any accommodation from occurring. Therefore, if the increase in minus sphere does not make the letters sharper, return to the previous position and leave the sphere there.

If the patient is not cyclopleged and is under 60 years old (ie, can accommodate), the duochrome test can be used to prevent over minusing. The duochrome is a slide that is displayed over the letters and makes the chart red on one side and green on the other. The patient is asked on which side are the letters clearest, the red or the green (or are they both the same?). If the green letters are clearer, then the patient may have more minus than he or she needs. Remove minus sphere (or add plus sphere) 0.25 D at a time until both sides are equal.

If the letters in the red are clearer, give minus sphere (or reduce plus sphere) 0.25 D at a time until both sides are equal.

Some examiners prefer; however, to leave their myopic patients "one click to the green." That is, they leave the patient with 0.25 D sphere more minus so that the letters on the green side are clearer, rather than having both sides equal.

Pinhole Disk

Most refractors have a pinhole disk as an accessory. It can be used to aid the examiner in cases when the patient's visual acuity does not meet expectations. By reducing the amount of

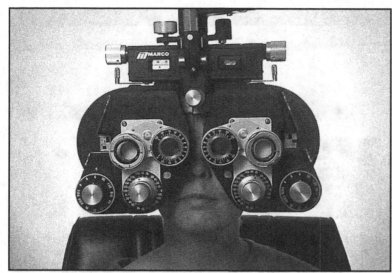

Figure 3-8. Rotary prism in binocular balancing. Three prism D base-up in front of the right eye, and 3 prism D base-down in front of the left eye. The right eye will see the higher image.

peripheral light, the pinhole disk reduces the refracting responsibility of the eye. Therefore, if a residual refractive error is present, the visual acuity should improve with the introduction of the pinhole disk. If this occurs, you should attempt to further refine the measurement until optimum vision is obtained. If no improvement is afforded, one can assume that the poor vision is due to nonoptical reasons.

Patients will often report that they can no longer see the eye chart when the pinhole disk is first placed in front of the eye. In this case, the examiner should encourage the patient to adjust his or her head position to align the pinhole with the visual axis.

Binocular Balance

The objective of binocular balancing is to ensure that the accommodation of both eyes is equally relaxed. Dissociation tests (those that cause a different image to be seen by each eye) are the most commonly used. The method will vary depending on whether or not the patient has the same visual acuity in both eyes. If the corrected vision is equal in both eyes, a comparison of the sharpness can be used. Otherwise, methods such as the duochrome test must be used.

Prism Dissociation Tests

Six D of vertical prism will cause the patient to see two charts, one above the other (or possibly diagonally if there is horizontal phoria present). Some examiners use the 6 prism diopter base-up auxiliary lens found in most refractors. However, this can sometimes lead to inaccuracy because the prism can detract from the quality of the image. Therefore, it is recommended that you use the Risley rotary prisms with 3.00 D base-down before the right eye and 3.00 D base-up before the left eye (Figure 3-8). The right eye will see the upper image.

Isolate the line of letters above the lowest line read. Ensure that the patient sees two separate lines (one for each eye). The patient is then asked to report if either line appears more sharp or distinct than the other. If the accommodative state is balanced, the patient will state that the lines are equal. However, this is not always the case.

Figure 3-9. Red/green duochrome test. This is an example of a target that may be used for red/green duochrome testing. Conventionally, red is shown on the patient's right (on this unit, red is on the left for use with a mirror system).

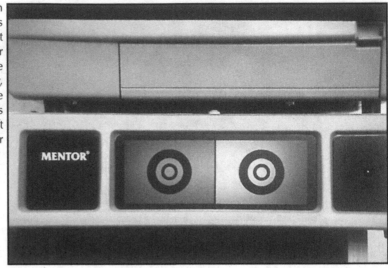

Figure 3-10. How light is refracted. Green light is refracted in front of red light. If white light is focused on the retina, green light should appear in front of the retina and red light behind it.

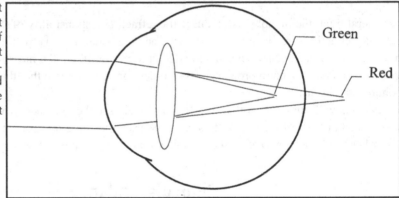

When the patient reports that one line is sharper, +0.25 sphere is added to the eye with the *more distinct* image. Again, the patient is asked to compare the two images for clarity. This step is repeated until both lines are equal, or the other image becomes more distinct (some examiners prefer to leave the dominant eye with the more distinct image if it is not possible to equalize the two eyes). Then the fog is slowly removed simultaneously from both eyes until maximal acuity is again achieved, taking care to not over minus.

Duochrome (Bichrome) Test

A slide that divides the chart into two sides, a red side and a green side (Figure 3-9), is used to perform the duochrome (or bichrome) test. The principle behind this test is the fact that green light waves are refracted more than red light waves (Figure 3-10). (Some examiners use the analogy of a green field in front of a red sunset to remember that green is refracted in front of red.)

The test begins with vertical prism (as described previously) and +0.50 D of fog in front of both eyes. This should position the focal point of all light in front of the retina. Since the red light is refracted the least, it is closest to the retina, causing the patient to report that the letters (or circles) on the red side appear sharper or more distinct than those on the green side.

Add -0.25 sphere and ask the patient to compare the two sides again. Continue towards the minus until both appear equal. Sometimes, the patient will report that with one lens the red side is sharper, then with an extra -0.25 sphere the green side is sharper. In this case, the author prefers to choose the lens that agrees with the original end point (the lens that the patient chose before beginning the duochrome test).

Some patients do not fully comprehend this test. Further explanation may be required to help the patient understand that it is the sharpness of the letters on each side that should be compared, not the contrast or blackness of them. Still, some patients will not be able to successfully complete the duochrome test.

Cycloplegic Refractometry   `OphT`

Arresting the accommodation of an eye using cycloplegic eye drops removes the variability in optical power caused by a contracting crystalline lens. This is especially useful on hyperopic patients who may not be able to fully relax their accommodation; the younger the patient, the more likely that latent hyperopia may exist. Cycloplegic refractometry is also indicated in children with esotropia because the strabismus may be accommodative in nature.

Various eye drops can be used to induce cycloplegia. Tropicamide, cyclopentolate, homatropine, and atropine are the most commonly used. Their differences lie in the speed and duration of action. When assessing the cycloplegic effect of a drop on a patient's eye, the examiner should ask the patient to read from a card held at a distance of 40 cm (16 in) while wearing the required corrective lenses for distance. If the cycloplegia is in full effect, the patient should not be able to read much better than Jaeger 10 (equivalent to 20/100). It should be noted that pupil dilation usually precedes and outlasts the cycloplegic effect.   `OptA`

Tropicamide is the shortest acting cycloplegic agent. Maximal effect occurs approximately 20 to 30 minutes after instillation and lasts for about 20 minutes (mydriasis will last 3 to 7 hours). Cyclopentolate has a stronger cycloplegic effect which will take 30 to 45 minutes to occur and will be maintained for about 30 to 45 minutes (mydriasis may linger for about 24 hours). Homatropine's maximal cycloplegia occurs in about 30 to 90 minutes and lasts for about 1 hour (mydriasis may last 6 hours to 4 days). Atropine is 10 times as potent as homatropine. It is usually instilled three times daily for 3 days prior to the exam, and then again 30 minutes before refractometry; the cycloplegic effect will last for 2 to 6 hours and the mydriatic effect for a few weeks.   `OptA`

The procedure for cycloplegic (wet) refractometry is essentially the same as that for manifest (dry) refractometry. Some accommodation may still be present, so the examiner should still push plus.

Alternate Procedures for Refining Astigmatism Correction

There will be times when the patient fails to respond accurately to the conventional methods of refining astigmatism. The examiner must then know other ways of determining the proper cylinder axis and power. One possibility is to use a hand-held cross cylinder of a greater power (such as 1.00 D). This is helpful for patients whose vision is not good enough to discern changes with a weaker cross cylinder. The process is the same as the refractor-mounted cross cylinder, with the exception that the examiner must be careful to keep the cross cylinder properly aligned. The handle is aligned with the correcting cylinder axis to refine the cylinder axis. When refining   `OphMT`

Figure 3-11. Astigmatic chart. Patient is asked to identify which of the four diamonds is sharpest. This allows the examiner to grossly determine axis of astigmatism.

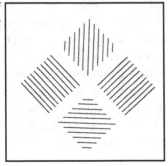

cylinder power, one of the colored lines (white or red) must be in alignment with the correcting cylinder axis.

Other techniques are discussed in the following sections.

Rotating Cylinder Axis

At times, the examiner may become discouraged and wish the patient could do his or her own measurement. While that may not be feasible, there is a variation to this wish; the patient's hand can be positioned on the knob that controls the cylinder axis and the patient is instructed to rotate it either way until he or she feels the vision is sharpest. This may not work very well if there is only 0.25 D of cylinder present. It would be permissible to increase the cylinder power up to 1.00 D or more for the purpose of this sequence (be sure to maintain the SE).

Four-Diamond Charts

The four-diamond charts are similar in concept to the astigmatic dial; parallel lines make up each diamond, and the lines in each diamond are oriented 45 degrees away from the neighboring diamonds (Figure 3-11). The degree of accuracy does not match the astigmatic dial since the axis can only be approximated to within about 20 degrees. Therefore, this test is usually used to determine if any astigmatism is present and, if so, the rough location of the axis. The procedure is the same as the astigmatic dial: fog by +0.50 D, ensure no cylinder power is in place, and then display the diamond. See the "Astigmatic Dial" section in the appropriate cylinder sign for information on determining the cylinder axis.

Stenopaic Slit

The stenopaic slit (alternative spelling: stenopeic) offers a method of performing refractometry on an individual with high or irregular astigmatism that may be present in conditions such as keratoconus. Light along one meridian passes through the slit while all other light is blocked. The examiner uses spheres to determine the best vision in each of the two primary meridians.

The first step is to create an adequate fog to position the conoid of Sturm in front of the retina. With the normal visual acuity chart displayed, the patient is asked to rotate the stenopaic slit until best vision is found. Assuming that the astigmatism is primarily in the cornea, the axis of the stenopaic slit should be coincident with the axis of the flattest keratometric measurement (minus cylinder axis). Ultimately, the first axis of the stenopaic slit is the minus cylinder axis.

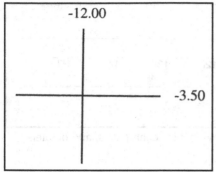

Figure 3-12. Power cross. Horizontal meridian measures -3.50, and vertical meridian measures -12.00.

However, the lens used to provide best vision at this position will be the spherical component of the net result.

The process of determining the sphere is the same as that used for conventional refractometry. The maximum amount of plus (or the least amount of minus) that provides the best vision is recorded using a power cross (Figure 3-12) along the axis of the stenopaic slit. In the example, the 180 degrees meridian had best vision with -3.50 sphere. The slit is then rotated 90 degrees and the process is repeated. In the example, the best vision at 90 degrees was achieved with -12.00 sphere.

Similar to manual lensometry, the difference between the two meridians is the cylindrical power. Using plus cylinder in our example, the net result would be -12.00 + 8.50 x 90. Remember that the maximum power of a cylinder is 90 degrees away from its axis; therefore, in our example, the axis is positioned at 90 degrees to correct the 180 degrees meridian. Net result for minus cylinder would be -3.50 -8.50 x 180.

Near Addition

Amplitude of Accommodation

Patients who have expressed a concern about the ability to read clearly should have their amplitude of accommodation measured (some examiners perform this test on all patients). Remember that a person should be corrected at near to provide twice as much accommodation than what is required to read at the desired distance. That is, if the patient wishes to read at 40 cm, 2.50 D of accommodation is used. This means the patient's amplitude of accommodation must be 5.00 D or more. This can be compared to lifting an object. If the object's weight is equal to the maximum that a person is able to lift, then the person's arms would become tired after a short while. However, if the person is capable of lifting an amount equal to twice the weight of the object, it would take more time for the person to tire. Similarly, if the patient has to exert maximum accommodation to read, clear focus cannot be maintained for very long.

Amplitude of accommodation is measured monocularly and binocularly. The monocular measurements should be similar. If a significant difference in amplitudes is found, the patient should be remeasured. Possible causes for a difference include an IOL implant in one eye, an error in determining the refractive error, or trauma.

The methods for determining amplitude of accommodation are described below. Once the amplitude of accommodation has been determined, it is possible to calculate the near addition (add) required for reading. Since it has been established that 50% of the amplitude should be held

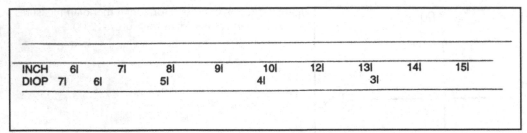

Figure 3-13. Reading rod. Markings on the reading rod show inches, centimeters, and diopters.

in reserve for comfortable reading, the following formula can be used: Addition = ND – (AA x 0.5), where ND equals the focusing power required to read at the desired distance, and AA is the patient's amplitude of accommodation. For example, if the patient wants to read at 40 cm, that would require 2.50 D (ND = 2.5). If the patient's amplitude of accommodation is 2.00 D (AA = 2.0), the near addition would be 1.50 D [2.5 – (2.0 x 0.5)].

Amplitude of accommodation is measured in diopters (how much accommodation the eye is able to exert). This is typically translated from the near POINT of accommodation which is measuring how far away from the eye focusing can be maintained—but one must keep in mind any uncorrected refractive error when calculating the amplitude. The range of accommodation is the distance between the near and far point of distinct vision; eg, a 2.00-D myope with 8.00 D of accommodation has a range of accommodation from 50 cm to 10 cm.

Push-up Method

Measuring the accommodative amplitude using the push-up method is done using the patient's distance correction. The patient is asked to indicate when fine print blurs as it is brought closer, and this distance is measured in centimeters. If the reading card of the refractor is used, the D value is indicated on the reading rod (Figure 3-13). If the print is blurred at 40 cm (16 in), plus sphere is added until the print is clear. The amount of sphere added is then subtracted from 2.50 (the amount of accommodation required at 40 cm). This method works well for patients over 40 years of age.

Minus Sphere Method

Fine print is positioned at 40 cm from the patient, and minus sphere lenses are added to the distance correction in 0.25 increments until the print blurs to the point where the patient cannot refocus. (The difference between the resulting measurement and the original, distant measurement is used.) Next, 2.50 D is added to this number to determine the amplitude of accommodation. For example, if the emmetrpoic (Plano) patient was able to maintain clarity using up to -3.00 D, the total amplitude of accommodation is 5.50 D (-3.00 + [-2.50]). The minus sign is disregarded when recording the amplitude because you have used minus sphere to neutralize a plus-powered entity: accommodation.

This method is especially useful in patients under 40 years.

Dynamic Cross Cylinder Test

The near add can be easily determined using a grid target and a cross cylinder (or the ±0.50 auxiliary lens on some refractors, see Figure 3-14). Before beginning the test, the patient's distance refractive error is corrected, and the grid target is positioned 40 cm from the patient. All lines on the grid should appear equal (clear or blurred). If one set of lines is sharper, it is likely that the astigmatism was not properly corrected; this must be rectified before continuing.

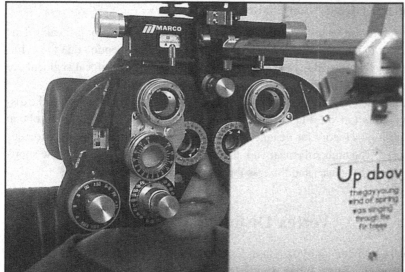

Figure 3-14. A ±0.50 auxiliary lens. Used in conjunction with the cross grid for determining if adequate accommodation is present.

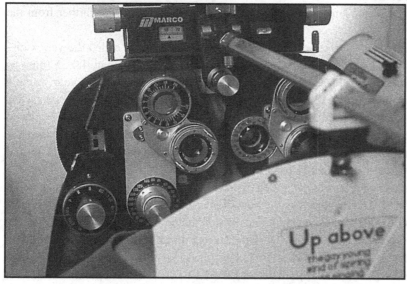

Figure 3-15. Cross cylinder for accommodation. An alternative to the ±0.50 auxiliary lens, the cross cylinder can be positioned with its minus cylinder axis at 90 degrees (regardless of correcting cylinder axis).

The cross cylinder is then introduced with its minus cylinder axis (red dot) at 90 degrees (regardless of where the correcting cylinder axis is located) (Figure 3-15). If the patient accommodates the proper amount for the distance of the grid target, all lines will appear equal, albeit slightly blurred. If the vertical lines appear clearer, the patient has over accommodated. Clearer horizontal lines mean the patient is not accommodating adequately. Some examiners remember this by imagining that the horizontal lines are arrows pointing to the optical shop next door (where the patient may purchase reading glasses/bifocals). Plus sphere lenses are added to the distance correction until all lines appear equal. This amount of additional plus indicates the bifocal add. If the patient would like single vision reading glasses, then the total lens power is used.

Adjusting Sphere for Best Near Vision

Some examiners prefer to use lenses to assess the need for reading glasses (or bifocals). This is done in a similar manner to that used for distance correction, with the exception that the cylinder component is not typically retested—the cylinder power and axis in the bifocal segment are the same as the distance portion. Therefore, only spheres are adjusted for near.

With the distance correction in place, the patient is instructed to hold the near target at the distance where he or she prefers to read. Plus sphere is added to the distance correction to obtain sharpness. Unlike the push plus theory for distance correction, the lowest addition that provides clear vision should be used. The higher the near add, the smaller the depth of focus (ie, the shorter the range in which objects are clear) and the less the patient will be satisfied.

Vertex Distance

If you have ever picked up a magnifying glass, you know that its power seems to change in relation to its distance from an object. When we use lenses to correct a moderate to high refractive error, we must take into account how far the lens is from the patient's eye for the same reason—the effective power of the lens changes as the lens is moved closer to or farther from the eye.

The distance from the back surface of a lens to the front of the eye is called the vertex distance. This distance should be measured whenever using lenses greater than 4.0 D (plus or minus). There are various vertex distance measuring devices on refractors; consult your owner's manual for instructions on their use. When measuring the vertex distance of a pair of spectacles, a distometer (caliper) should be used. The arm of the caliper with a flattened surface is placed against the closed eyelid, and the plunger is depressed until the other caliper arm is against the back surface of the lens. Distometers are calibrated to take into account the thickness of a normal eyelid. The vertex distance is read directly from the scale.

To calculate the power of a lens at any given distance, the following formula can be used: $N = 1 \div (1 \div D - [VD1 - VD2])$ where N is the new diopter power, D is the power of the lens, VD1 is the existing vertex distance (in meters), and VD2 is the new vertex distance (in meters). For example, suppose you have a -8.00 lens (D) with a vertex distance of 6 mm (VD1), and you would like to know what power would be required to have the same effect at a distance of 13 mm (VD2). $N = 1 \div (1 \div -8.0 - [0.006 - 0.013])$; therefore, $N = 1 \div (-0.125 -[-0.007])$; $N = 1 \div -0.118$; $N = -8.47$. In other words, a -8.47-D lens would be required at 13 mm to have the same effect as a -8.00-D lens at 6 mm.

There are charts available to convert effective powers from one vertex distance to another. The most common reason for doing this is when converting a spectacle prescription to contact lens power, or vice versa. If the power of the lens is 4 D or more (plus or minus), vertex distance must be concidered. For example, a -4.25 spectacle correction at 12 mm would only need to be -4.00 D for a contact lens. On the plus side, a +4.25 spectacle correction at 12 mm would need to be a +4.50 contact lens. The difference in power between the contact lens and spectacle lens increases proportionately with the refractive error.

Table 3-1.
Comparison of Visual Acuity and Refractive Errors

Myopia	Expected Acuity
-0.50	20/25—20/30
-1.00	20/40
-1.50	20/60
-2.00	20/100
-3.00	20/200—20/300
-4.00	20/400

Correlating Refractive Error with Visual Acuity

The unaided visual acuity of a myopic person should correlate to the amount of myopia present (Table 3-1). This is a useful guide to help the examiner evaluate the possibility of over minusing a patient. One must be observant when assessing unaided acuity because some patients will attempt to squint to provide better vision.

Latent Nystagmus

Some patients are prone to nystagmus when one eye is covered (latent nystagmus). This can pose a problem for the examiner since an eye with constant movement will have decreased vision. Therefore, the fellow eye must not be occluded. Granted, this would make decision-making difficult for the patient as lenses are changed since the vision in one eye remains the same. Removing the occluder is still possible, however. A high-powered plus sphere lens (+8.00 over the estimated refractive error) is used to blur the vision of the fellow eye. Since the eye is not actually occluded, the latent nystagmus is resolved, and the vision is blurred to the extent that the chart cannot be read.

Spectacles of Refractometry (The Return of the Glasses)

Despite the best efforts to prescribe the ideal combination of lenses for a patient, some people will return to the office with a frown on their face and their new spectacles in their hand. There is a seemingly infinite number of reasons why patients are not happy with their new glasses. It could be that the lenses were made incorrectly, a different base curve was used, or a significant change in lens power is not tolerated, to name just a few. This section will briefly describe a systematic approach to help isolate the cause of the patient's unhappiness.

The first and probably the simplest step is to measure the power of the lenses using a lensometer. Compare the measurements to what was prescribed. There should be less than 0.25 D difference in power of sphere or cylinder, and the cylinder axis should be within a couple of degrees. (Remember that those individuals with high amounts of astigmatism cannot tolerate *any* error in cylinder axis.)

In most cases, the power of the lenses matches the prescription provided. So, the search for the problem continues. Mark the optical centers of each lens using the lensometer. Compare the patient's interpupillary distance with the distance between the optical center of the lenses. If the lenses have any significant power, the induced prism caused by incorrectly positioned optical centers can cause troubling symptoms (eg, a pulling sensation whenever the glasses are worn or the vague sensation that the glasses "aren't right").

In the case of bifocals, assess the position of the upper edge of the bifocal segment while the patient is wearing the glasses. The rule of thumb is that the top of the bifocal segment should be aligned with the lower eyelid margin. Bifocals that are too low will cause problems because the patient's head is tilted back to move the segment high enough to read. When the segment is positioned too high, the patient may have visual symptoms (a blur inferiorly) or complain that the head must be tilted downward in order to see distant objects clearly.

If the mystery has not yet been solved, then it is time to go to the examination room to repeat the measurement of the refractive error. The process may take longer than usual since the original measurement may not have produced the proper result. If different values are found for the refractive error, then a decision must be made regarding whether the difference is sufficient to cause the patient's symptoms. However, as is often the case, the result is the same as (or very close to) the previous attempt. This can leave the examiner scratching his or her head, wondering where the problem could be.

There are certain scenarios in which, despite all the proper measurements being done, the patient will have symptoms causing complaints. This situation can sometimes be avoided if the patient is warned ahead of time about what to expect with the new glasses and how long the symptoms can be expected to last. Trying to explain this to the patient *after* hearing his or her complaints is almost futile. The patient will perceive these explanations as a feeble attempt to avoid fixing the problem. Therefore, any time a prescription is given for a pair of glasses where the parameters do not match the existing pair, the patient should be informed that the new glasses may feel a bit strange for a couple of days or possibly even weeks. Problems that persist after a couple of weeks should be investigated.

The common situations that cause temporary problems are:
- Prescribing more plus for a hyperope than what was measured with manifest refractometry (but not necessarily the entire cycloplegic amount).
- Changing the cylindrical axis, especially when it is moved farther away from 90 or 180 degrees.
- Increasing the cylinder power.
- Changing the base curve and/or material of the lens.

References

Appleton B. *Clinical Optics.* Thorofare, NJ: SLACK Incorporated; 1990.

Brooks C, Borish I. *System for Ophthalmic Dispensing.* 2nd ed. Newton, Mass: Butterworth-Heinemann; 1996.

Cassin B. *Fundamentals for Ophthalmic Medical Personnel.* Philadelphia, Pa: WB Saunders; 1995.

Copeland JC. *Streak Retinoscopy.* Chicago, Ill: Stereo Optical Incorporated; 1990.

Duane TD, Jaeger EA. *Biomedical Foundations of Ophthalmology.* Philadelphia, Pa: Lippincott-Raven Publishers; 1996.

Grosvenor T. *Primary Care Optometry.* 3rd ed. Newton, Mass: Butterworth-Heinemann; 1996.

Ledford J. *Exercises in Refractometry.* Thorofare, NJ: SLACK Incorporated; 1990.

Stein H, Slatt B, Stein R. *The Ophthalmic Assistant.* 6th ed. St Louis, Mo: CV Mosby; 1994.

Vaughan D, Asbury T, Riordan-Eva R. *General Ophthalmology.* 14th ed. Norwalk, Conn: Appleton and Lange; 1995.

Appendix A

The Metric System

The metric system is a system for measuring length, weight, and volume. It is used in most English-speaking countries although its acceptance in the United States has been slow.

The beauty of the metric system lies in the fact that it is based on multiples of 10. In addition, the same prefixes indicating fractions of units can be applied to all three types of measurements.

The base metric unit for length is the meter. The gram (g) is the base for weight and the liter (L) is the base for volume. Table A-1 shows the prefixes that are most useful in the eyecare field. These prefixes can be combined to any of the base units. For example, the terms kilometer (km), kilogram (kg), and kiloliter (kL) refer to 103 of their respective units (ie, 1000 m, gm, or L).

The metric system is widely used in the scientific community, including the eyecare field. Because of this, most of the formulas used in optics are written to use metric units. If your measurements are taken in nonmetric units (eg, inches, pounds, or fluid ounces), you will need to be able to convert them to metric units in order to work the formula. Table A-2 gives common conversions.

It is also important to note that while measurements may be given in the metric system, the formula may call for a different fraction unit. For example, the formula for focal length is $D = 1 \div F$ where D is the power of the lens in diopters and F is the focal length in meters. However, you may be given the focal length in centimeters. It is important to know the formula and to read the question carefully in order to be sure that you are working with the correct units. If not, it is easy to go from one unit to the other by moving the decimal point accordingly.

At times, it may also be necessary to be able to convert visual acuity measurements from those based on 20 feet to those based on the metric system (6 m is standard). Table A-3 gives these conversions.

Table A-1
Metric Fraction Prefixes

Prefix	Part of Base Unit
Kilo	10^3 OR base unit X 1000
Hecto	10^2 OR base unit X 100
Deci	10^{-1} OR base unit X 0.1
Centi	10^{-2} OR base unit X 0.01
Milli	10^{-3} OR base unit X 0.001
Micro	10^{-6} OR base unit X 0.000001

Table A-2
Metric Equivalents

1 centimeters	0.3937 inch (centimeters X 0.3937 = inches)
1 inch	2.54 centimeters (inches X 2.54 = centimeters)
1 meters	39.37 inches (meters X 39.37 = inches)
1 yard	0.9144 meters (yards X 0.9144 = meters)
1 cubic centimeter	0.061 inch^3 (cubic centimeters X 0.061 = inches^3)
1 cubic inch	16.39 cc (cubic inches X 16.39 = cc)
1 ounce	28.3 grams (ounces X 28.3 = grams)
1 liter	2.11 pints (liters X 2.11 = pints)
1 gallon	3.79 liters (gallons X 3.79 = liters)
1 gram	0.035 ounces (grams X 0.035 = ounces)
1 pound	28.3 grams (pounds X 28.3 = grams)
1 kilogram	2.2 pounds (kilograms X 2.2 = pounds)

Table A-3
Visual Acuity

Based on 20 Feet	Based on 6 Meters
20/400	6/120
20/300	6/90
20/200	6/60
20/100	6/30
20/80	6/24
20/70	6/21
20/60	6/18
20/50	6/15
20/40	6/12
20/30	6/9
20/25	6/7.5
20/20	6/6
20/15	6/4.5
20/10	6/3

Appendix B

Abbreviations

Common Abbreviations in Optics

General

R	right
L	left
OD	right eye
OS	left eye
OU	both eyes
↑	increase
↓	decrease
Δ	change
Rx	prescription

Visual Acuity

VA	visual acuity
DA	distant acuity
NA	near acuity
BVA	best visual acuity
c̄c̄	with correction
s̄c̄	without correction
PH	pinhole
CF	count fingers
HM	hand motion
LPr	light projection
LP	light perception
NLP	no light perception
J	Jaeger
P	point

Lensometry

NW	now wearing (patient's present glasses *Rx*)
add	addition
segs	segments
BF/bi	bifocal
TF/tri	trifocal
sph	sphere
cyl	cylinder
°	degree
X	axis
Δ	prism diopter
BU	base-up
BD	base-down
BI	base-in
BO	base-out
DBC	distance between centers

OCS	optical center separation (same as DBC)
DBL	distance between lenses
UV	ultraviolet
cm	centimeters
mm	millimeters

Contact Lenses

HCL	hard contact lens
SCL	soft contact lens
EWCL	extended wear contact lens
GPCL/GP	gas permeable contact lens
DW	daily wear

Refractometry

PD	pupillary distance
IPD	interpupillary distance (same as PD)
MR	manifest refractometry
CR	cycloplegic refractometry
AR	autorefraction
GR	gross retinoscopy
NR	net retinoscopy
accom	accommodation
OR	over-refractometry
VD	vertex distance
BC	base curve
AK	astigmatic keratotomy
e-LASIK	epithelial laser-assisted in-situ keratomileusis
epi-LASIK	epithelial laser-assisted in-situ keratomileusis
LASEK	laser epithelial keratomileusis
LASIK	laser-assisted in-situ keratomileusis
PRK	photorefractive keratectomy
RK	radial keratotomy

Appendix C

Exercises

The Case Option Exercises

by Janice K. Ledford, COMT

How to Use the Case Option Exercises

The Case Option Directory lists the various types of optical cases on which you may choose to work. Exercises in Unit One let you choose the patient's responses and then tell you the appropriate optical action that corresponds to that response. This is the equivalent of watching a refractometrist at work and having him or her explain what he or she is doing as the test goes along.

Unit Two puts you in the examiner's chair. This time you are given the patient's response. You must then choose which of the options is the most correct action. If you make an incorrect choice, the text explains why. If you make a good judgment, your selection will be reinforced, and you move on through the measurement by choosing new responses.

Of course, the array of real patient responses is unlimited (and sometimes strange, misleading, or downright malingering). I have attempted to keep the choices and results within reasonable and believable limits.

The exercise pages are coded so you can "practice" in whichever cylinder you choose. A minus (–) sign denotes minus cylinder, and a plus (+) sign denotes plus cylinder.

The first frame of each case gives you the patient's present glasses prescription (if worn), visual acuity with that prescription, and sometimes other pertinent information. You must always start at frame #1 of a case. From there, follow the frame numbers of the options you choose.

The exercises are arranged in an easily understood format (see sample frame on page 87). Each exercise is identified by a lowercase letter. The frame number and exercise letter appear in the upper-left corner of each frame. When working an exercise, be sure to follow THESE frame numbers.

Beneath the frame number and exercise letter are bold face numbers that identify the lenses in the refractor at that point. Boldface numbers within the text of a frame show the refractor readings after a change has been made. This feature ensures that you will not "get lost" as you go from frame to frame.

The numbers in the upper right of the frame show you what frame you just came from to help you keep your place. Occasionally there may be more than one possibility as the options branch and regroup, but when following the options, follow the frame numbers on the upper left.

The abbreviations appearing in the exercises were explained previously in Appendix B.

To get maximum benefit from the exercises, work them in order and go through each one more than once, choosing different options when appropriate.

Protocol for the Exercises

The Exercises are written using the following protocol for refractometry.

- Regardless of cylinder sign, when dealing with sphere power, plus is *always* offered first.

- If the patient accepts more minus sphere, the next step is to have him or her read again from the chart. If he or she cannot read smaller letters than before, return to the previous sphere setting. This is to avoid over minusing.

- Start with the chart on a line or two *larger* than what the patient read when you checked visual acuity. There is no need for him or her to struggle with reading the chart at the beginning of the test. (You will push for smaller letters later.)

- Always check cylinder axis and power with the eye chart on one or two lines larger than the patient's best vision.

- When using the astigmatic dial, fog with +0.50 more than the spherical refraction currently in the phoroptor. Ask patient if any of the lines on the "clock face" are darker, sharper, or clearer than the others. If so, ask which lines (eg, running from 12:00 to 6:00 or from 2:00 to 8:00). To find the axis in plus cylinder, multiply the smaller "clock hour" by 30 and rotate by 90 degrees. To find the axis in minus cylinder, multiply the smaller "clock hour" by 30. For either cylinder type, crank in 0.25 cyl until patient says all lines are equally dark.

- When using the astigmatic dial, after selecting the axis and adding cylinder, you must adjust the sphere. In plus cylinder, give –0.25 sphere for each +0.50 D of cylinder power you gave. In minus cylinder, give +0.25 sphere for each –0.50 D of cylinder power.

- When using the cross cylinder to refine axis and power, if the patient says that the two choices are about the same, it means that you are currently on the right setting. (This is because you are straddling the correct point, and each choice is an equal distance from that point.)

I.   Gross Spheres—Offered in 0.50-D steps, starting with plus. Continue until the vision blurs, then return to the previous setting. You may offer minus only if the first +0.50 step blurs the vision. If more minus does not improve the vision by helping the patient to read smaller letters, return to the previous sphere setting.

II.   Cylinder Axis—*Always* refine the axis before refining the power. In plus cylinder, follow the white dot. In minus cylinder, follow the red dot. Move in 15-degree steps until the patient reverses direction. (Smaller increments may be used with higher cylinder powers.) Then move in increasingly smaller steps (eg, 7 degrees, then 3 degrees) until both choices look the same.

III.   Cylinder Power—Start with 0.50-D steps. In plus cylinder, if the patient chooses the white dot, add more plus cylinder. If the patient chooses the red dot, reduce plus cylinder. In minus cylinder, if the patient chooses the red dot, give more minus cylinder. If the patient chooses the white dot, reduce the amount of minus cylinder. With either cylinder power, once the patient reverses his or her choice (ie, has been asking for less but now wants more), try 0.25 steps until both choices look the same. Remove the cross cylinder and have the patient read the smallest letters that he or she is able to see.

IV.   Fine Spheres—Again, always offer plus first. Work in 0.25-D steps. Give plus until the chart blurs; then return to the setting prior to where the blurring occurred. If the patient takes minus, he or she must earn it by reading smaller letters on the chart. If he or she cannot do this, return to the previous setting. Record the measurement and the vision obtained with it.

Case Option Exercises Directory

Unit One. Astigmatism With Glasses

Unit Two. Unknown Refractive Error (Astigmatic Dial Option)

Sample Frame

Exercise Frame #

Preceding Frame #

Present
Phoropter
Setting

Phoropter
Settings After
Change

Text

Options

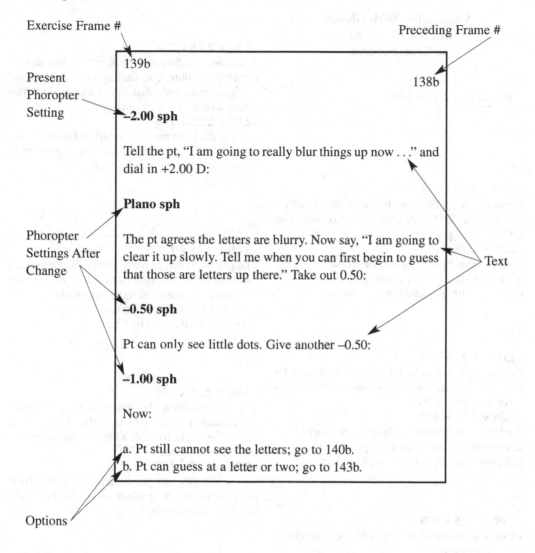

139b

138b

−2.00 sph

Tell the pt, "I am going to really blur things up now . . ." and dial in +2.00 D:

Plano sph

The pt agrees the letters are blurry. Now say, "I am going to clear it up slowly. Tell me when you can first begin to guess that those are letters up there." Take out 0.50:

−0.50 sph

Pt can only see little dots. Give another −0.50:

−1.00 sph

Now:

a. Pt still cannot see the letters; go to 140b.
b. Pt can guess at a letter or two; go to 143b.

Unit One

Astigmatism With Glasses
PLUS CYLINDER
a. Gross Spheres

1a
NW: −2.50 + 2.25 x 178
VA c̄ 20/60
Go to 2a.

2a
                                              1a
−2.50 + 2.25 x 178
Chart is on 20/60, which the pt reads with a few misses. To begin with gross spheres, you offer 0.50 of plus first:
−2.00 + 2.25 x 178
Ask, "Is this better (pause) or worse?"
a. Pt says this is more clear; go to 3a.
b. Pt says this is more blurred; go to 4a.

3a
                                              2a
−2.00 + 2.25 x 178
Pt has accepted 0.50 more plus. You wonder how much more plus the pt will take. So you offer another +0.50:
−1.50 + 2.25 x 178
And ask, "Is this more clear . . . or blurry?"
a. Pt says this is more clear; go to 5a.
b. Pt says this is more blurred; go to 6a.

4a
                                              2a
−2.00 + 2.25 x 178
Pt says addition of 0.50 has blurred the chart, so you return to:
−2.50 + 2.25 x 178
then try 0.50 of minus:
−3.00 + 2.25 x 178
and ask, "Is this more clear . . . or blurry?"
a. Pt says more clear; go to 7a.
b. Pt says they look about the same; go to 8a.

5a
                                              3a
−1.50 + 2.25 x 178
Pt has accepted yet more plus. You are dubious but wisely offer yet another +0.50:
−1.00 + 2.25 x 178
a. Pt says this is about the same; go to 9a.
b. Pt says this has blurred; go to 10a.

6a
                                              3a
−1.50 + 2.25 x 178
Addition of 0.50 more plus sphere has caused the chart to blur. You realize you have passed the maximum plus that the pt can accept. You return to the previous setting:
−2.00 + 2.25 x 178
and ask the pt to read the smallest line of letters possible. The pt reads 20/30. You are ready to begin checking the astigmatism.
Go to 15a.

7a
                                              4a
−3.00 + 2.25 x 178
The pt has asked for more minus. Since you are cautious about handing out minus, you ask the pt to read the smallest letters possible.
a. Pt still reads 20/60; go to 11a.
b. Pt reads 20/30; go to 12a.

8a
                                              4a
−3.00 + 2.25 x 178
The pt says that the addition of 0.50 more minus does not really change the clarity of the chart. You want to push as much plus as possible and restore the +0.50:
−2.50 + 2.25 x 178
Gross spheres has produced no change from the starting *Rx*. You are ready to begin checking the astigmatism.
Go to 16a.

9a
                                              5a
−1.00 + 2.25 x 178
Pt has accepted another +0.50 plus, stating that the chart has not changed. You are dubious but want to give as much plus as possible. So you offer yet another +0.50:
−0.50 + 2.25 x 178
which the pt says is blurry. You know you have pushed as much plus as possible and return to the previous setting:
−1.00 + 2.25 x 178
You now ask the pt to read the smallest letters possible.
a. Pt still reads 20/60; go to 13a.
b. Pt reads 20/30; go to 14a.

10a

5a

−1.00 + 2.25 x 178

Pt states last addition of 0.50 has blurred the chart. You know you have pushed as much plus as possible and return to the previous setting:

−1.50 + 2.25 x 178

You now ask the pt to read the smallest letters possible, and the pt reads 20/40. You are ready to begin checking the astigmatism.

Go to 15a.

11a

7a

−3.00 + 2.25 x 178

The pt can read no better now than with the pt's original *Rx* . . . gross changes in sphere have not improved the pt. You want to leave the pt with the maximum amount of plus possible and return to your original reading:

−2.50 + 2.25 x 178

You are ready to check the pt's astigmatism.

Go to 16a.

12a

7a

−3.00 + 2.25 x 178

The pt's vision has improved substantially, but it is still not 20/20. Adding more minus fails to improve the pt's vision further. You are ready to check the pt's astigmatism.

Go to 15a.

13a

9a

−1.00 + 2.25 x 178

The pt has taken a large change in sphere yet shows no improvement. You are suspicious and decide to try −0.50 again:

−1.50 + 2.25 x 178

Now the pt says this is clearer, and the pt proves it by reading 20/40. You are ready to check the pt's astigmatism.

Go to 15a.

14a

9a

−1.00 + 2.25 x 178

Pt has made a substantial improvement in acuity although it required a sizable addition of plus. You are ready to check the pt's astigmatism.

Go to 15a.

15a

You have completed the gross spheres step with a reasonable amount of change and a reasonable improvement in vision. You now have several options:

a. Move on to Refine Cylinder Axis Exercise b, PLUS CYLINDER; go to 1b.

b. Start this Exercise again, and choose different options; go to 1a.

16a

You have completed the gross spheres step although the pt's vision has not improved. You still hope to increase the pt's acuity by working with the cylinder axis and power. You now have several options:

a. Move on to Refine Cylinder Axis Exercise b, PLUS CYLINDER; go to 1b.

b. Start this Exercise again, and choose different options; go to 1a.

+

Astigmatism With Glasses
PLUS CYLINDER
b. Refine Cylinder Axis

1b

Beginning *Rx*: −2.50 + 2.25 x 178
After gross spheres (for a common starting place):
−2.00 + 2.25 x 178
Suppose the pt has read 20/30 with this MR. You now want letters that you know the pt can see easily and put the 20/50 line up. You swing the cross cylinder into place and align the turnstile with the axis. The white dot is counterclockwise to 178, and the red dot is clockwise. You tell the pt, "You are looking at the letters through glass #1 right now. Which seems better, #1 here . . . (pause, then flip cross cylinder over) . . . or this #2?"
a. Pt says #1 is better; go to 2b.
b. Pt says #2 is better; go to 4b.
c. Pt says they are about the same; go to 6b.

2b

1b

−2.00 + 2.25 x 178
Pt says #1 is clearer. You turn the cross cylinder back to choice #1 and note that the white dot is counterclockwise to 178. So, you rotate the axis 15 degrees counterclockwise toward the white dot:
−2.00 + 2.25 x 013
The white dot is still counterclockwise to 013. You say, "Which is clearer now . . . this #3 . . . (pause, flip) . . . or #4?"
a. Pt says #4; go to 3b.
b. Pt says they are about the same; go to 7b.

3b

2b

−2.00 + 2.25 x 013
The pt has chosen #4, with the white dot clockwise to 013. Thus, you will move back toward the axis that you originally came from. You rotate this axis clockwise halfway between 013 and 178:
−2.00 + 2.25 x 006
The white dot is now clockwise to 006. You ask the pt, "Which is better here . . . this #5 that you are looking at now . . . (pause, flip) . . . or this #6?" Pt says they look the same. You are through with axis and ready to check cylinder power.
Go to 9b.

4b

1b

−2.00 + 2.25 x 178
Pt has chosen #2, in which the white dot is clockwise to 178. You rotate toward the white dot 15 degrees clockwise:
−2.00 + 2.25 x 163
The white dot is still clockwise to 163. You say, "Which is clearer now . . . this #3 . . . (pause, flip) . . . or #4?"
a. Pt says #4; go to 5b.
b. Pt says they are about the same; go to 8b.

5b

4b

−2.00 + 2.25 x 163
The pt has chosen #4, with the white dot counterclockwise to 163. This is back toward the direction you originally came from. You rotate the axis counterclockwise halfway between 163 and 178:
−2.00 + 2.25 x 171
The white dot is still counterclockwise to 171. You ask the pt. "Which is better here . . . this #5 that you are looking at now . . . (pause, flip) . . . or this #6?" The pt hesitates. You realize that this probably means that #5 and #6 look about the same. So you ask, "Or do they look about the same?" Pt says they look the same. You are through with axis and ready to check cylinder power.
Go to 9b.

6b

1b

−2.00 + 2.25 x 178
Pt has said both choices look the same. You realize that this indicates that the axis is now correct, and you are ready to check cylinder power.
Go to 9b.

7b

2b

−2.00 + 2.25 x 013
Pt has said both choices look the same. You realize that this indicates that the axis is now correct, and you are ready to check cylinder power.
Go to 9b.

8b

4b

−2.00 + 2.25 x 163

Pt has said both choices look the same. You realize that this indicates that the axis is now correct, and you are ready to check cylinder power.

Go to 9b.

9b

You have completed the refine cylinder axis step. Your options are the following:

a. Move on to Refine Cylinder Power Exercise c, PLUS CYLINDER; go to 1c.

b. Start this Exercise again, and choose different options; go to 1b.

c. Call your mother to complain about what a pain studying is.

Astigmatism With Glasses
PLUS CYLINDER
c. Refine Cylinder Power

1c

Beginning *Rx*: –2.50 + 2.25 x 178, VA c̄ 20/60
After gross spheres:
–2.00 + 2.25 x 178, VA c̄ 20/30
After refining cylinder axis (for a common starting place):
–2.00 + 2.25 x 171
You are now ready to check cylinder power. You rotate the cross cylinder so that the "P" is in line with the axis. To help you keep your place, each choice is followed by a "W" for the white dot or an "R" for the red dot . . . whichever is showing at "P." You ask, "Which is clearer now . . . this #7(W) . . . (pause, flip). . . or #8(R)?"
a. Pt says #7 is better; go to 2c.
b. Pt says #8 is better; go to 6c.
c. Pt says they are about the same; go to 12c.

2c

1c

–2.00 + 2.25 x 171
Pt says #7, when the white dot appeared, is clearer. You realize this means you should add some more PLUS cylinder power. You give 0.50:
–2.00 + 2.75 x 171
You flip the cross cylinder so that the white dot is again on "P" and ask, "Which is clearer here . . .#9(W) . . . (pause, flip) . . . or #10(R)?"
a. Pt says #10; go to 3c.
b. Pt says they are about the same; go to 11c.

3c

2c

–2.00 + 2.75 x 171
Pt has chosen red dot this time, so you know you should reduce the cylinder power. You remove 0.25, which is half of the 0.50 that you added in the last step:
–2.00 + 2.50 x 171
The red dot is still up. You ask, "Which is better now . . . this #11(R) . . . (pause, flip) . . . or #12(W)?"
a. Pt says #11 is better; go to 4c.
b. Pt says they are about the same; go to 5c.

4c

3c

–2.00 + 2.50 x 171
Pt has again chosen the red dot. You remove another 0.25, which returns you to your starting point:
–2.00 + 2.25 x 171
That is fine. The pt would probably continue to go back and forth between +2.25 cyl and +2.50 cyl all day. You want the pt to have the least amount of cylinder possible. You are now ready for fine spheres.
Go to 13c.

5c

3c

–2.00 + 2.50 x 171
The pt says that the lenses look the same. You realize you have reached your end point and are ready for fine spheres.
Go to 13c.

6c

1c

–2.00 + 2.25 x 171
The pt has chosen #8, with the red dot showing at "P." You realize this means you should reduce the cyl power. You take out 0.50:
–2.00 + 1.75 x 171
The red dot is still on "P." You ask, "Which is clearer now . . . this #9(R) . . . (pause, flip) . . . or #10(W)?"
a. Pt chooses #10; go to 7c.
b. Pt says they are about the same; go to 10c.

7c

6c

–2.00 + 1.75 x 171
The pt has chosen #10, with the white dot at "P." You know you should restore some of the cyl power you took out previously. You add back 0.25, which is half of the 0.50 that you took out before:
–2.00 + 2.00 x 171
The white dot is still at "P." You ask, "Which seems better now . . . this #11(W) . . . (pause, flip) . . . or #12(R)?"
a. Pt chooses #11; go to 8c.
b. Pt says they are the same; go to 9c.

8c

7c

−2.00 + 2.00 x 171
The pt has requested another addition of cyl power. You give another 0.25, which returns you to your starting point:
−2.00 + 2.25 x 171
That is fine. The pt would probably continue to go back and forth between +2.00 cyl and +2.25 cyl all day. You want the pt to have the least amount of cyl possible. You are ready for fine spheres.
Go to 13c.

9c

7c

2.00 + 2.00 x 171
The pt says that the lenses look the same. You realize you have reached your end point and are ready for fine spheres.
Go to 13c.

10c

6c

−2.00 + 1.75 x 171
The pt says that the lenses look the same. You realize you have reached your end point and are ready for fine spheres.
Go to 13c.

11c

2c

−2.00 + 2.75 x 171
The pt says that the lenses look the same. You realize you have reached your end point and are ready for fine spheres.
Go to 13c.

12c

1c

−2.00 + 2.25 x 171
The pt says that the lenses look the same. You realize you have reached your end point and are ready for fine spheres.
Go to 13c.

13c
You have completed the Refine Cylinder Power step and now have several options:
a. Continue this refractometric measurement into Fine Spheres Exercise d, PLUS CYLINDER; go to 1d.
b. Start this Exercise over, choosing different options; go to 1c.
c. Refry your beans for the Mexican dinner you are planning.

+

Astigmatism With Glasses
PLUS CYLINDER
d. Fine Spheres

1d
Beginning *Rx*: −2.50 + 2.25 x 178, VA c̄ 20/60
After gross spheres:
−2.00 + 2.25 x 178, VA c̄ 20/30
After refining cylinder axis:
−2.00 + 2.25 x 171
After refining cylinder power (for a common starting place):
−2.00 + 2.25 x 171
You are now ready to check for fine spheres. You rotate the cross cylinder out of the way. Now it is time to see if the cylinder changes you made helped the pt's acuity, so you ask the pt to read the smallest letters possible.
a. Pt reads 20/25; go to 2d.
b. Pt reads 20/40; go to 5d.

2d

1d

−2.00 + 2.25 x 171
Pt has read 20/25. You now begin the fine spheres stage by offering 0.25 more plus (always offer plus first):
−1.75 + 2.25 x 171
and ask, "Can you see the letters any better now?"
a. Pt says they are about the same; go to 3d.
b. Pt says letters are a bit blurred now; go to 15d.
c. Pt says letters are a bit clearer; go to 16d.

3d

2d, 14d

−1.75 + 2.25 x 171
The pt says the letters are about the same. You still want to give the most plus you can and offer an additional 0.25:
−1.50 + 2.25 x 171
The pt reports this has blurred the chart, so you take the 0.25 back out:
−1.75 + 2.25 x 171
Your refractometric measurement is complete. Now is the time to urge your pt to read the smallest letters possible.
a. Pt reads 20/30; go to 4d.
b. Pt reads 20/20; go to 17d.

4d

3d

−1.75 + 2.25 x 171
The pt does not read as well now as when you started the fine spheres test. Although the pt said that the letters seemed the same in frame 2d, something is amiss. You try going back 0.25 again:
−2.00 + 2.25 x 171
Pt now reads 20/20⁻. You are through!
Final MR: −2.00 + 2.25 x 171
VA c̄ 20/20⁻
Go to 22d.

5d

1d

−2.00 + 2.25 x 171
The pt reads less now than before you checked the pt's astigmatism. Before moving into fine spheres, you want to know if the change in astigmatic correction caused the decrease in acuity. With the pt looking at the 20/40 letters, you ask, "Are the letters more clear like they are now . . . (pause, then turn the axis back to 178 degrees) . . . or here?"
−2.00 + 2.25 x 178
a. Pt notes no difference; go to 6d.
b. Pt says letters are clearer now; go to 13d.
c. Pt detects slight blur now; go to 14d.

6d

5d

−2.00 + 2.25 x 178
The pt says the letters look the same at axis 171 as 178. You like to change things as little as possible, so you leave the refractor at this setting and ask the pt to read again. The pt manages 20/30. You now move into fine spheres and start by offering 0.25 more plus (always try plus first):
−1.75 + 2.25 x 178
a. Pt says this is better; go to 7d.
b. Pt says this is about the same; go to 12d.

7d

6d, 13d

−1.75 + 2.25 x 178

Pt says the addition of 0.25 more plus is clearer. You want to give the maximum amount of plus possible, so you offer yet another 0.25:

−1.50 + 2.25 x 178

The pt reports that this has blurred the chart, so you take the 0.25 back out:

−1.75 + 2.25 x 178

Your refractometry is finished. Now, you want the pt to read the smallest letters possible.

a. Pt reads 20/30; go to 8d.

b. Pt reads 20/20; go to 11d.

8d

7d

−1.75 + 2.25 x 178

The pt reads no better now than when you started fine spheres. Just to be sure, you take out the 0.25:

−2.00 + 2.25 x 178

and ask again, "Is this still about the same?"

a. Pt says this is better; go to 9d.

b. Pt says about the same; go to 10d.

9d

8d

−2.00 + 2.25 x 178

Pt now says this is better. So you push the pt to read the smallest letters possible. The pt reads 20/20⁻. You are through!

Final MR: −2.00 + 2.25 x 178

VA c̄ 20/20⁻

Go to 22d.

10d

8d

−2.00 + 2.25 x 178

Pt says this is still the same. Since you want to push plus, you restore the 0.25:

−1.75 + 2.25 x 178

and ask the pt to read one more time. The pt reads 20/25⁻. You are through!

Final MR: −1.75 + 2.25 x 178

VA c̄ 20/25⁻

Go to 22d.

11d

7d

−1.75 + 2.25 x 178

Pt has read 20/20, so you are finished!

Final MR: −1.75 + 2.25 x 178

VA c̄ 20/20

Go to 22d.

12d

6d, 13d

−1.75 + 2.25 x 178

The pt says the letters are about the same. You still want to give the most plus you can and offer an additional 0.25:

−1.50 + 2.25 x 178

The pt reports this has blurred the chart, so you take the 0.25 back out:

−1.75 + 2.25 x 178

You are almost through! You urge the pt to read the smallest letters possible. The pt reads 20/20⁻.

Final MR: −1.75 + 2.25 x 178

VA c̄ 20/20⁻

Go to 22d.

13d

5d

−2.00 + 2.25 x 178

The pt maintains that the pt's original axis is clearer than that found in the refining axis step. You have the pt prove it by asking him or her to read smaller letters on the chart. The pt reads 20/30. You now move into fine spheres. You start by offering 0.25 more plus (always try plus first):

−1.75 + 2.25 x 178

a. Pt says this is better; go to 7d.

b. Pt says this is about the same; go to 12d.

14d

5d

−2.00 + 2.25 x 178
The pt says that the letters are a bit blurred now. So you return to the axis of 171:
−2.00 + 2.25 x 171
and urge the pt to read again. This time, the pt manages 20/30. You now begin fine spheres by offering 0.25 more plus (always offer plus first):
−1.75 + 2.25 x 171
and ask, "Are the letters any clearer now?"
a. Pt says letters are a bit blurred now; go to 15d.
b. Pt says letters are about the same; go to 3d.

15d

2d, 14d

−1.75 + 2.25 x 171
The pt says the letters are blurred now, so you know you have pushed beyond the maximum plus. You remove the 0.25:
−2.00 + 2.25 x 171
Now try −0.25:
−2.25 + 2.25 x 171
The pt says this is no better. Since there was no improvement and you want to give the most plus you can, you restore the 0.25:
−2.00 + 2.25 x 171
and urge the pt to read the smallest letters possible. The pt reads 20/25+. You are through!
Final MR: −2.00 + 2.25 x 171
VA c̄ 20/25+
Go to 22d.

16d

2d

−1.75 + 2.25 x 171
Pt has said the letters are clearer. You want to give the maximum amount of plus possible, so you offer yet another 0.25:
−1.50 + 2.25 x 171
a. Pt says this is blurred; go to 18d.
b. Pt says this is about the same; go to 19d.

17d

3d

−1.75 + 2.25 x 171
The pt has read 20/20 with the above measurement. You are through!
Final MR: −1.75 + 2.25 x 171
VA c̄ 20/20
Go to 22d.

18d

16d

−1.50 + 2.25 x 171
The pt says the letters are blurred now, so you know you have pushed beyond maximum plus. You remove the 0.25:
−1.75 + 2.25 x 171
and urge the pt to read the smallest letters possible. The pt reads 20/20. You are finished!
Final MR: −1.75 + 2.25 x 171
VA c̄ 20/20
Go to 22d.

19d

16d

−1.50 + 2.25 x 171
Pt says the letters look about the same. You still want to give the most plus you can and offer an additional 0.25:
−1.25 + 2.25 x 171
The pt reports this has blurred the chart, so you take the 0.25 back out:
−1.50 + 2.25 x 171
Now you urge the pt to read the smallest letters possible.
a. Pt reads 20/20⁻, go to 20d.
b. Pt reads 20/30⁻, go to 21d.

20d

19d

−1.50 + 2.25 x 171
You are through!
Final MR: −1.50 + 2.25 x 171
VA c̄ 20/20⁻
Go to 22d.

21d

19d

−1.50 + 2.25 x 171
The pt does not read as well as before you started the fine spheres test. Although the pt thought the letters seemed clearer in frame 16d, something is wrong. You try going back 0.25 again:
−1.75 + 2.25 x 171
Now the pt again reads 20/25+. You are through!
Final MR: −1.75 + 2.25 x 171
VA c̄ 20/25+
Go to 22d.

22d

You now have several alternatives:

a. Start this Exercise again, and make different choices; go to 1d.

b. Return to the Directory, and choose another Exercise.

c. Restring your ukulele.

**Astigmatism With Glasses
MINUS CYLINDER
a. Gross Spheres**

1a
NW: –2.50 – 2.25 x 088
VA c̄ 20/60
Go to 2a.

2a

1a

–2.50 – 2.25 x 088
Chart is on 20/60, which the pt reads with a few misses. To begin with gross spheres, you offer 0.50 of plus first:
–2.00 – 2.25 x 088
Ask, "Is this better (pause) or worse?"
a. Pt says this is more clear; go to 3a.
b. Pt says this is more blurred; go to 4a.

3a

2a

–2.00 – 2.25 x 088
Pt has accepted 0.50 more plus. You wonder how much more plus the pt will take. So you offer another +0.50:
–1.50 – 2.25 x 088
And ask, "Is this more clear . . . or blurry?"
a. Pt says this is more clear; go to 5a.
b. Pt says this is more blurred; go to 6a.

4a

2a

–2.00 – 2.25 x 088
Pt says addition of 0.50 has blurred the chart, so you return to:
–2.50 – 2.25 x 088
then try 0.50 of minus:
–3.00 – 2.25 x 088
and ask, "Is this more clear . . . or blurry?"
a. Pt says more clear; go to 7a.
b. Pt says they look about the same; go to 8a.

5a

3a

–1.50 – 2.25 x 088
Pt has accepted yet more plus. You are dubious, but wisely offer yet another +0.50:
–1.00 – 2.25 x 088
a. Pt says this is about the same; go to 9a.
b. Pt says this has blurred; go to 10a.

6a

3a

–1.50 – 2.25 x 088
Addition of 0.50 more plus sphere has caused the chart to blur. You realize you have passed the maximum plus that the pt can accept. You return to the previous setting:
–2.00 – 2.25 x 088
and ask the pt to read the smallest line of letters possible. The pt reads 20/30. You are ready to begin checking the astigmatism.
Go to 15a.

7a

4a

–3.00 – 2.25 x 088
The pt has asked for more minus. Since you are cautious about handing out minus, you ask the pt to read the smallest letters possible.
a. Pt still reads 20/60; go to 11a.
b. Pt reads 20/30; go to 12a.

8a

4a

–3.00 – 2.25 x 088
The pt says that the addition of 0.50 more minus does not really change the clarity of the chart. You want to push as much plus as possible and restore the +0.50:
–2.50 – 2.25 x 088
Gross spheres has produced no change from the starting *Rx*. You are ready to begin checking the astigmatism.
Go to 16a.

9a

5a

–1.00 – 2.25 x 088
Pt has accepted another +0.50 plus, stating that the chart has not changed. You are dubious but want to give as much plus as possible. So you offer yet another +0.50:
–0.50 – 2.25 x 088
which the pt says is blurry. You know you have pushed as much plus as possible and return to the previous setting:
–1.00 – 2.25 x 088
You now ask the pt to read the smallest letters possible.
a. Pt still reads 20/60; go to 13a.
b. Pt reads 20/30; go to 14a.

10a
                                          5a
–1.00 – 2.25 x 088
Pt states last addition of 0.50 has blurred the chart. You know you have pushed as much plus as possible and return to the previous setting:
–1.50 – 2.25 x 088
You now ask the pt to read the smallest letters possible, and the pt reads 20/40. You are ready to begin checking the astigmatism.
Go to 15a.

11a
                                          7a
–3.00 – 2.25 x 088
The pt can read no better now than with the pt's original *Rx* . . . gross changes in sphere have not improved the pt. You want to leave the pt with the maximum amount of plus possible and return to your original reading:
–2.50 – 2.25 x 088
You are ready to check the pt's astigmatism.
Go to 16a.

12a
                                          7a
–3.00 – 2.25 x 088
The pt's vision has improved substantially, but it is still not 20/20. Adding more minus fails to improve pt's vision further. You are ready to check the pt's astigmatism.
Go to 15a.

13a
                                          9a
–1.00 – 2.25 x 088
The pt has taken a large change in sphere yet shows no improvement. You are suspicious and decide to try –0.50 again:
–1.50 – 2.25 x 088
Now the pt says this is clearer and proves it by reading 20/40. You are ready to check the pt's astigmatism.
Go to 15a.

14a
                                          9a
–1.00 – 2.25 x 088
Pt has made a substantial improvement in acuity although it required a sizable addition of plus. You are ready to check the pt's astigmatism.
Go to 15a.

15a
You have completed the gross spheres step with a reasonable amount of change and a reasonable improvement in vision. You now have several options:
a. Move on to Refine Cylinder Axis Exercise b, MINUS CYLINDER; go to 1b.
b. Start this Exercise again, and choose different options; go to 1a.

16a
You have completed the gross spheres step, although the pt's vision has not improved. You still hope to increase the pt's acuity by working with the cylinder axis and power. You now have several options:
a. Move on to Refine Cylinder Axis Exercise b, MINUS CYLINDER; go to 1b.
b. Start this Exercise again, and choose different options; go to 1a.

—

**Astigmatism With Glasses
MINUS CYLINDER
b. Refine Cylinder Axis**

1b

Beginning *Rx*: −2.50 − 2.25 x 088
After gross spheres (for a common starting place):
−2.00 − 2.25 x 088
Suppose the pt has read 20/30 with this MR. You now want letters that you know the pt can see easily and put the 20/50 line up. You swing the cross cylinder into place and align the turnstile with the axis. The red dot is counterclockwise to 088, and the white dot is clockwise. You tell the pt, "You are looking at the letters through glass #1 right now. Which seems better, #1 here . . . (pause, then flip cross cylinder over) . . . or this #2?"
a. Pt says #1 is better; go to 2b.
b. Pt says #2 is better; go to 4b.
c. Pt says they are about the same; go to 6b.

2b

1b

−2.00 − 2.25 x 088
Pt says #1 is clearer. You turn the cross cylinder back to choice #1 and note that the red dot is counterclockwise to 088. So you rotate the axis 15 degrees counterclockwise toward the red dot:
−2.00 − 2.25 x 103
The red dot is still counterclockwise to 103. You say, "Which is clearer now . . . this #3 . . . (pause, flip) . . . or #4?"
a. Pt says #4; go to 3b.
b. Pt says they are about the same; go to 7b.

3b

2b

−2.00 − 2.25 x 103
The pt has chosen #4, with the red dot clockwise to 103. Thus you will move back toward the axis that you originally came from. You rotate the axis clockwise halfway between 103 and 088:
−2.00 − 2.25 x 096
The red dot is now clockwise to 096. You ask the pt: "Which is better here . . . this #5 that you are looking at now . . . (pause, flip) . . . or this #6?" Pt says they look the same. You are through with axis and ready to check cylinder power.
Go to 9b.

4b

1b

−2.00 − 2.25 x 088
Pt has chosen #2, in which the red dot is clockwise to 088. You rotate toward the red dot 15 degrees clockwise:
−2.00 − 2.25 x 073
The red dot is still clockwise to 073. You say, "Which is the clearer now . . . this #3 . . . (pause, flip) . . . or #4?"
a. Pt says #4; go to 5b.
b. Pt says they are about the same; go to 8b.

5b

4b

−2.00 − 2.25 x 073
The pt has chosen #4, with the red dot counterclockwise to 073. This is back toward the direction you originally came from. You rotate the axis counterclockwise halfway between 073 and 088:
−2.00 − 2.25 x 081
The red dot is still counterclockwise to 081. You ask the pt, "Which is better here . . . this #5 that you are looking at now . . . (pause, flip) . . . or this #6?" The pt hesitates. You realize that this probably means that #5 and #6 look about the same. So you ask, "Or do they look about the same?" Pt says they look the same. You are through with axis and ready to check cylinder power.
Go to 9b.

6b

1b

−2.00 − 2.25 x 088
Pt has said both choices look the same. You realize that this indicates that the axis is now correct, and you are ready to check cylinder power.
Go to 9b.

7b

2b

−2.00 − 2.25 x 103
Pt has said both choices look the same. You realize that this indicates that the axis is now correct, and you are ready to check cylinder power.
Go to 9b.

8b

4b

–2.00 – 2.25 x 073
Pt has said both choices look the same. You realize that this indicates that the axis is now correct, and you are ready to check cylinder power.
Go to 9b.

9b
You have completed the refine cylinder axis step. Your options are the following:
a. Move on to Refine Cylinder Power Exercise c, MINUS CYLINDER; go to 1c.
b. Start this Exercise again, and choose different options; go to 1b.
c. Call your mother to complain about what a pain studying is.

Astigmatism With Glasses
MINUS CYLINDER
c. Refine Cylinder Power

1c

Beginning *Rx*: –2.50 – 2.25 x 088, VA c̄ 20/60
After gross spheres:
–2.00 – 2.25 x 088, VA c̄ 20/30
After refining cylinder axis (for a common starting place):
–2.00 – 2.25 x 081
You are now ready to check cylinder power. You rotate the cross cylinder so that the "P" is in line with the axis. To help you keep your place, each choice is followed by an "R" for the red dot or a "W" for the white dot . . . whichever is showing at "P." You ask, "Which is clearer now . . . this #7(R) . . . (pause, flip) . . . or #8(W)?"
a. Pt says #7 is better; go to 2c.
b. Pt says #8 is better; go to 6c.
c. Pt says they are about the same; go to 12c.

2c

1c

–2.00 – 2.25 x 081
Pt says #7, when the red dot appeared, is clearer. You realize this means you should add some MINUS cylinder power. You give 0.50:
–2.00 – 2.75 x 081
You flip the cross cylinder so that the red dot is again on "P" and ask, "Which is clearer here . . . #9(R) . . . (pause, flip) . . . or #10(W)?"
a. Pt says #10; go to 3c.
b. Pt says they are about the same; go to 11c.

3c

2c

–2.00 – 2.75 x 081
Pt has chosen white dot this time, so you know you should reduce the amount of minus cylinder power. You remove 0.25, which is half of the 0.50 that you added in the last step:
–2.00 – 2.50 x 081
The white dot is still up. You ask, "Which is better now . . . this #11(W) . . . (pause, flip) . . . or #12(R)?"
a. Pt says #11 is best; go to 4c.
b. Pt says they are about the same; go to 5c.

4c

3c

–2.00 – 2.50 x 081
Pt has again chosen the white dot. You remove another 0.25, which returns you to your starting point:
–2.00 – 2.25 x 081
That is fine. The pt would probably continue to go back and forth between –2.25 cyl and –2.50 cyl all day. You want the pt to have the least amount of cylinder possible. You are now ready for fine spheres.
Go to 13c.

5c

3c

–2.00 – 2.50 x 081
The pt says that the lenses look the same. You realize you have reached your end point and are ready for fine spheres.
Go to 13c.

6c

1c

–2.00 – 2.25 x 081
The pt has chosen #8, with the white dot showing at "P." You realize this means you should reduce the cylinder power. You take out 0.50:
–2.00 – 1.75 x 081
The white dot is still on "P." You ask, "Which is clearer now . . . this #9(W) . . . (pause, flip) . . . or#10(R)?"
a. Pt chooses #10; go to 7c.
b. Pt says they are about the same; go to 10c.

7c

6c

–2.00 – 1.75 x 081
The pt has chosen # 10, with the red dot at "P." You know you should restore some of the cyl power you took out previously. You give back –0.25, which is half of the 0.50 that you gave before:
–2.00 – 2.00 x 081
The red dot is still at "P." You ask, "Which seems better now . . . this #11(R) . . . (pause, flip) . . . or #12(W)?"
a. Pt chooses #11; go to 8c.
b. Pt says they are the same; go to 9c.

8c

7c

–2.00 – 2.00 x 081

The pt has requested another addition of minus cyl power. You give another 0.25, which returns you to your starting point:

–2.00 – 2.25 x 081

That is fine. The pt would probably continue to go back and forth between –2.00 cyl and –2.25 cyl all day. You want the pt to have the least amount of cylinder possible. You are ready for fine spheres.

Go to 13c.

9c

7c

–2.00 – 2.00 x 081

The pt says that the lenses look the same. You realize you have reached your end point and are ready for fine spheres.

Go to 13c.

10c

6c

–2.00 – 1.75 x 081

The pt says that the lenses look the same. You realize you have reached your end point and are ready for fine spheres.

Go to 13c.

11c

2c

–2.00 – 2.75 x 081

The pt says that the lenses look the same. You realize you have reached your end point and are ready for fine spheres.

Go to 13c.

12c

1c

The pt says that the lenses look the same. You realize you have reached your end point and are ready for fine spheres.

Go to 13c.

13c

You have completed the Refine Cylinder Power step, and now have several options:

a. Continue this refractometric measurement into Fine Spheres Exercise d, MINUS CYLINDER; go to 1d

b. Start this Exercise over, choosing different options; go to 1c.

—

Astigmatism With Glasses
MINUS CYLINDER
d. Fine Spheres

1d

Beginning *Rx*: –2.50 – 2.25 x 088, VA c̄ 20/60
After gross spheres:
–2.00 + 2.25 x 088, VA c̄ 20/30
After refining cylinder axis:
–2.00 + 2.25 x 081
After refining cylinder power (for a common starting place):
–2.00 + 2.25 x 081
You are now ready to check for fine spheres. You rotate the cross cylinder out of the way. Now it is time to see if the cylinder changes you made helped the pt's acuity, so you ask the pt to read the smallest letters possible.
a. Pt reads 20/25; go to 2d.
b. Pt reads 20/40; go to 5d.

2d

1d

–2.00 – 2.25 x 081
Pt has read 20/25. You now begin the fine spheres stage by offering 0.25 more plus (always offer plus first):
–1.75 – 2.25 x 081
and ask, "Can you see the letters any better now?"
a. Pt says they are about the same; go to 3d.
b. Pt says letters are a bit blurred now; go to 15d.
c. Pt says letters are a bit clearer; go to 16d.

3d

2d, 14d

–1.75 – 2.25 x 081
The pt says the letters are about the same. You still want to give the most plus you can, and offer an additional 0.25:
–1.50 – 2.25 x 081
The pt reports this has blurred the chart, so you take the plus back out:
–1.75 – 2.25 x 081
Your refractometric measurement is complete. Now is the time to urge your pt to read the smallest letters possible.
a. Pt reads 20/30; go to 4d.
b. Pt reads 20/20; go to 17d.

4d

3d

–1.75 – 2.25 x 081
The pt does not read as well now as when you started the fine spheres test. Although the pt said that the letters seemed the same in frame 2d, something is wrong. You try going back 0.25 again:
–2.00 – 2.25 x 081
Pt now reads 20/20⁻. You are through!
Final MR: –2.00 – 2.25 x 081
VA c̄ 20/20⁻
Go to 22d.

5d

1d

–2.00 – 2.25 x 081
The pt reads less now than before you checked the pt's astigmatism. Before moving into fine spheres, you want to know if the change in astigmatic correction caused the decrease in acuity. With the pt looking at the 20/40 letters, you ask, "Are the letters more clear as they are now . . . (pause, then turn the axis back to 088 degrees) or here?"
–2.00 – 2.25 x 088
a. Pt notes no difference; go to 6d.
b. Pt says letters are clearer now; go to 13d.
c. Pt detects slight blur now; go to 14d.

6d

5d

–2.00 – 2.25 x 088
The pt says the letters look the same at axis 081 as 088. You like to change things as little as possible, so you leave the refractor at this setting and ask the pt to read again. The pt manages 20/30. You now move into fine spheres, and start by offering 0.25 more plus (always try plus first):
–1.75 – 2.25 x 088
a. Pt says this is better; go to 7d.
b. Pt says this is about the same; go to 12d.

7d

6d, 13d

–1.75 – 2.25 x 088
Pt says the addition of 0.25 more plus is clearer. You want to give the maximum amount of plus possible, so you offer yet another 0.25:
–1.50 – 2.25 x 088
The pt reports that this has blurred the chart, so you take the 0.25 back out:
–1.75 – 2.25 x 088
Your refractometry is finished. Now, you want the pt to read the smallest letters possible.
a. Pt reads 20/30; go to 8d.
b. Pt reads 20/20; go to 11d.

8d

7d

–1.75 – 2.25 x 088
The pt reads no better now than when you started fine spheres. Just to be sure, you take out the 0.25:
–2.00 – 2.25 x 088
and ask again, "Is this still about the same?"
a. Pt says this is better; go to 9d.
b. Pt says about the same; go to 10d.

9d

8d

–2.00 – 2.25 x 088
Pt now says this is better. So you push the pt to read the smallest letters possible. The pt reads 20/20⁻. You are through!
Final MR: –2.00 – 2.25 x 088
VA c̄ 20/20⁻
Go to 22d.

10d

8d

–2.00 – 2.25 x 088
Pt says this is still the same. Since you want to push plus, you restore the 0.25:
–1.75 – 2.25 x 088
and ask the pt to read one more time. The pt reads 20/25⁻. You are through!
Final MR: –1.75 – 2.25 x 088
VA c̄ 20/25⁻
Go to 22d.

11d

7d

–1.75 – 2.25 x 088
Pt has read 20/20, so you are finished!
Final MR: –1.75 – 2.25 x 088
VA c̄ 20/20
Go to 22d.

12d

6d, 13d

–1.75 – 2.25 x 088
The pt says the letters are about the same. You still want to give the most plus you can, and offer an additional 0.25:
–1.50 – 2.25 x 088
The pt reports this has blurred the chart, so you take the 0.25 back out:
–1.75 – 2.25 x 088
You are almost through! You urge the pt to read the smallest letters possible. The pt reads 20/20⁻.
Final MR: –1.75 – 2.25 x 088
VA c̄ 20/20⁻
Go to 22d.

13d

5d

–2.00 – 2.25 x 088
The pt maintains that the pt's original axis is clearer than that found in the refining axis step. You have the pt prove it by asking him or her to read smaller letters on the chart. The pt reads 20/30. You now move into fine spheres. You start by offering 0.25 more plus (always try plus first):
–1.75 – 2.25 x 088
a. Pt says this is better; go to 7d.
b. Pt says this is about the same; go to 12d.

14d

5d

−2.00 − 2.25 x 088
The pt says that the letters are a bit blurred now. So you return to the axis of 081:
−2.00 − 2.25 x 081
and urge the pt to read again. This time, the pt manages 20/30. You now begin fine spheres by offering 0.25 more plus (always offer plus first):
−1.75 − 2.25 x 081
and ask, "Are the letters any clearer now?"
a. Pt says letters are a bit blurred now; go to 15d.
b. Pt says letters are about the same; go to 3d.

15d

2d, 14d

−1.75 − 2.25 x 081
The pt says the letters are blurred now, so you know you have pushed beyond maximum plus. You remove the 0.25:
−2.00 − 2.25 x 081
Now try −0.25:
−2.25 − 2.25 x 081
The pt says this is no better. Since there was no improvement and you want to give the most plus you can, you restore the 0.25:
−2.00 − 2.25 x 081
and urge the pt to read the smallest letters possible. The pt reads 20/25⁺. You are through!
Final MR: −2.00− 2.25 x 081
VA c̄ 20/25⁺
Go to 22d.

16d

2d

−1.75 − 2.25 x 081
Pt has said the letters are clearer. You want to give the maximum amount of plus possible, so you offer yet another 0.25:
−1.50 − 2.25 x 081
a. Pt says this is blurred; go to 18d.
b. Pt says this is about the same; go to 19d.

17d

3d

−1.75 − 2.25 x 081
The pt has read 20/20 with the above measurement. You are through!
Final MR: −1.75 − 2.25 x 081
VA c̄ 20/20
Go to 22d.

18d

16d

−1.50 − 2.25 x 081
The pt says the letters are blurred now, so you know you have pushed beyond maximum plus. You remove the 0.25:
−1.75 − 2.25 x 081
and urge the pt to read the smallest letters possible. The pt reads 20/20. You are finished!
Final MR: −1.75 − 2.25 x 081
VA c̄ 20/20
Go to 22d.

19d

16d

−1.50 − 2.25 x 081
Pt says the letters look about the same. You still want to give the most plus you can, and offer an additional 0.25:
−1.25 − 2.25 x 081
The pt reports this has blurred the chart, so you take the 0.25 back out:
−1.50 − 2.25 x 081
Now you urge the pt to read the smallest letters possible.
a. Pt reads 20/20⁻, go to 20d.
b. Pt reads 20/30⁻, go to 21d.

20d

19d

−1.50 − 2.25 x 081
You are through!
Final MR: −1.50 − 2.25 x 081
VA c̄ 20/20⁻
Go to 22d.

21d

19d

−1.50 − 2.25 x 081
The pt does not read as well as before you started the fine spheres test. Although the pt thought the letters seemed clearer in frame 16d, something is wrong. You try going back 0.25 again:
−1.75 − 2.25 x 081
Now the pt again is reading 20/25⁺. You are through!
Final MR: −1.75 − 2.25 x 081
VA c̄ 20/25⁺
Go to 22d.

22d
You now have several alternatives:
a. Start this Exercise again, and make different choices; go to 1d.
b. Return to the Directory, and choose another Exercise.
c. Restring your ukulele.

Unit Two

e. Unknown Refractive Error
PLUS CYLINDER

1e

NW: none
VA s̄ 20/200
Go to 2e.

2e

1e

Plano sph
You place the empty refractor to the pt. The chart is on:
a. 20/200; go to 3e.
b. 20/400; go to 4e.
c. 20/100; go to 5e.

3e

2e

Plano sph
No, it is better to start with letters a bit larger than the pt's starting acuity.
Go back to 2e, and try again.

4e

2e

Plano sph
Right. Ordinarily you would start at about two lines larger than the pt's starting acuity. But many charts do not have anything between 20/200 and 20/400. So, 20/400 will have to do.
Go to 6e.

5e

2e

Plano sph
No, these are too small. You want to start with letters a bit larger than the pt's starting acuity.
Go back to 2e, and try again.

6e

4e

Plano sph
The pt affirms he or she can see the 20/400 letter. You are ready to start gross spheres. You first offer:
a. +0.25: **+0.25 sph**; go to 7e.
b. +0.50: **+0.50 sph**; go to 8e.
c. −0.50: **−0.50 sph**; go to 9e

7e

6e

+0.25 sph
Offering plus first is right, but gross spheres goes in 0.50-D steps, remember?
Go back to 6e, and try again.

8e

6e

+0.50 sph
Right! Gross spheres uses 0.50 steps, and you should always offer plus first. Next you should:
a. Add another 0.50: **+1.00 sph**; go to 10e.
b. Ask the pt if the chart is clearer; go to 11e.

9e

6e

−0.50 sph
No, always offer plus first.
Go back to 6e, and try again.

10e

8e

+1.00 sph
No, first you need to find out if the power change is helping or not.
Go back to 8e, and try again.

11e

8e

+0.50 sph
Yes, you should ask if the pt notes any improvement after each plus change during gross spheres. In this case, the pt reports that the 20/400 letter is a bit clearer. Next you should:
a. Continue to add 0.50 steps of plus, assessing each change until pt reports blurring; go to 12e.
b. Ask the pt how far down on the chart he or she can read now; go to 13e.

+

12e

11e

+0.50 sph

This is a good method for gross spheres . . . provided that the pt is taking plus. When the pt reports blurring, simply go 0.50 D back to the previous setting, then have the pt read the smallest letters possible.

Of course, this is inappropriate when working in a minus direction, where the pt must 'earn' more minus by reading smaller letters.

Go to 14e.

13e

11e

+0.50 sph

There is nothing wrong with having the pt read the chart. But when adding plus, it is quicker to move ahead in +0.50 steps until the pt reports blurring. At that point, simply go back 0.50 to the previous setting; then have the pt read the smallest letters possible.

Of course, this method is inappropriate when working in a minus direction.

Go to 14e.

14e

12e, 13e

+0.50 sph

After going through all that, let us suppose that the pt says that the letters are more blurred. You dutifully remove the +0.50:

Plano sph

Next you try giving:

a. −0.25: **−0.25 sph**; go to 15e.

b. −0.50: **−0.50 sph**; go to 16e.

15e

14e

−0.25 sph

No, gross spheres works in 0.50-D steps.

Go back to 14e, and try again.

16e

14e

−0.50 sph

Yes. You are still in gross spheres and using 0.50-D steps. The pt says this is clearer. Next you:

a. Offer another −0.50: **−1.00 sph**; go to 17e.

b. Have the pt read smaller letters; go to 18e.

17e

16e

−1.00 sph

Well, while it is true that a 0.50-D step probably will not take the pt from 20/200 to 20/20, it is best to be cautious when offering minus.

Go back to 16e, and choose again.

18e

16e

−0.50 sph

Right. When the pt takes minus, the pt should earn it by reading smaller letters with each change.

Go to 19e.

19e

18e

−0.50 sph

Let us suppose that the pt says that the 20/200 is clearer but still cannot read 20/100. Next you should:

a. Check for astigmatism; go to 20e.

b. Offer more minus; go to 21e.

20e

19e

−0.50 sph

No, you are jumping the gun a bit. Although this may be the most minus the pt should have, you should offer more minus this time because the pt's acuity is still so poor. The next 0.50 change may yield 20/100.

Go back to 19e, and choose again.

21e

19e

−0.50 sph

Yes, you should offer more minus. The pt's poor acuity may take a substantial amount of minus to improve it. So you try another −0.50:

−1.00 sph

and the pt reads 20/100. In fact, you continue in −0.50 steps and the pt reads smaller letters each time for TWO more steps:

−2.00 sph

Now the pt reads 20/60. You give yet another −0.50:

−2.50 sph

The pt says this is better, but still reads only 20/60.

Next you:

a. Go back 0.50: **−2.00 sph**; go to 22e.

b. Offer another −0.50: **−3.00 sph**; go to 23e

22e.

21e

–2.00 sph

This is fine. You are sure you have not over minused this way. If the pt needs more minus, he or she will pick it up in fine spheres. (The other choice was okay, too.) You are ready to check for astigmatism.

Go to 26e.

23e

21e

–3.00 sph

This is fine. (The other choice was okay, too.) In this case, the pt still cannot read more than 20/60. Now you should return to:

a. **–2.50 sph**; go to 24e.
b. **–2.00 sph**; go to 25e.

24e

23e

–2.50 sph

No, you did not go back far enough. The last TWO changes (a total of 1.00) did not produce any improvement, and you want the least minus possible.

Go back to 23e, and choose again.

25e

23e

–2.00 sph

Right. The last TWO changes (a total of 1.00) did not produce any improvement, and you want the least minus possible. You are now ready to check for astigmatism.

Go to 26e.

26e

22e, 25e

–2.00 sph

You are going to use the astigmatic dial to detect astigmatism. You show the pt the dial and ask:

a. Are there any lines that are darker than the rest? Go to 27e.
b. Are any of the lines more blurred than the rest? Go to 28e.

27e

26e

–2.00 sph

Right. You need to know if there are darker lines. If the pt says all the lines look the same, what do you do next?

a Go directly to fine spheres; go to 29e.
b. Add +0.50: **–1.50 sph**; go to 30e.

28e

26e

–2.00 sph

No, you need to identify the darker lines.

Go back to 26e, and try again.

29e

27e

–2.00 sph

No, you are not ready for fine spheres yet. If all the lines look the same, add 0.50 of plus:

–1.50 sph

If astigmatism is present, this maneuver will usually bring it out.

Go to 30e.

30e

27e, 29e

–1.50 sph

Right. The addition of 0.50 of plus will often bring out the darker lines. Suppose the pt now says that the lines running from 1 o'clock across to 7 o'clock are darker. Where do you set your axis?

a. 060 degrees; go to 31e.
b. 120 degrees; go to 32e.

31e

30e

-1.50 +   x 060

No, you need to review the "rule of 30."

Go back to 30e, and choose again.

32e

30e

-1.50 +   x 120

Right. Using the "rule of 30," multiply the smaller clock hour by 30 and rotate by 90 degrees. In this case, 1 o'clock is smaller; 1 x 30 = 30 + 90 = 120. Your next step is to:

a. Add cyl power until all lines seem equal; go to 33e.
b. Go back to the eye chart, flip down the cross cyl, and get busy; go to 34e.

33e

32e

−1.50 +   x 120

Right. Now suppose the lines seem equal after 0.50 D of cyl is added:

−1.50 + 0.50 x 120

Next you should:

a. Remove the 0.50 of plus you used to identify the astigmatism: **−2.00 +0.50 x 120**; go to 35e

b. Give −0.25 sphere power for each +0.50 D of cyl power you used: **−1.75 + 0.50 x 120**; go to 36e.

34e

32e

−1.50 +   x 120

No, not yet. You need to determine about how much cyl power the pt needs.

Go back to 32e, and try again.

35e

33e

−2.00 + 0.50 x 120

No. You need to adjust the sphere according to how much cyl you used.

Go back to 33e, and choose again.

36e

33e

−1.75 + 0.50 x 120

Right! Go to 37e.

37e

36e

−1.75 + 0.50 x 120

Now you are ready to return to the letter chart. What size letters do you choose to begin the cross cyl stage? (Last acuity was 20/60.)

a. 20/80; go to 38e.

b. 20/60; go to 39e.

c. 20/40; go to 40e.

38e

37e

−1.75 + 0.50 x 120

Right. The 20/80 line is two lines above the acuity after gross spheres. During cross cyl refinement, you want to use letters that you know the pt can see. Now, you pop the cross cyl into place. How do you line it up to check the axis?

a. "P" in line with the axis; go to 41e.

b. Turnstile in line with axis; go to 42e.

39e

37e

−1.75 + 0.50 x 120

No. 20/60 is the pt's acuity after gross spheres. You need something easier to see.

Go back to 37e, and choose again.

40e

37e

−1.75 + 0.50 x 120

No. This is even smaller than the pt's acuity after gross spheres. You need letters that the pt can see easily.

Go back to 37e, and choose again.

41e

38e

−1.75 + 0.50 x 120

No, the "P" is for power refinement.

Go back to 38e, and try again.

42e

38e

−1.75 + 0.50 x 120

Yes. The turnstile is aligned with the axis when you refine axis position. Suppose the white dot is clockwise to your 120 degree axis. You now ask, "Which is clearer, this #1. . . (pause, flip) . . . or #2." The pt says #2 is clearer. Which way do you rotate the axis now?

a. Clockwise 15 degrees: **−1.75 + 0.50 x 105**; go to 43e.

b. Counterclockwise 15 degrees: **−1.75 + 0.50 x 135**, go to 44e.

43e

42e

−1.75 + 0.50 x 105

No, you should follow the white dot. When you flipped the cross cyl over for choice #2, this placed the white dot counterclockwise from the turnstile.

Go back to 42e, and try again.

44e

42e

−1.75 + 0.50 x 135
Right. You realized that flipping the cross cyl over for choice #2 placed the white dot counterclockwise to the turnstile, where it remains. You now say, "And now which seems better, this #3 . . . (pause, flip) . . . or #4?" The pt chooses #3. Where do you rotate the axis now?
a. Clockwise 15 degrees: **−1.75 + 0.50 x 120**; go to 45e.
b. Counterclockwise 15 degrees: **−1.75 + 0.50 x 150**; go to 46e.

45e

44e

1.75 + 0.50 x 120
No. The pt chose #3, which had the white dot in a counterclockwise direction. You should follow the white dot.
Reread frame 44e, and choose again.

46e

44e

−1.75 + 0.50 x 150
Yes. During choice #3, the white dot was counterclockwise from the turnstile. Following the white dot 15 degrees counterclockwise brought you to 150 degrees. Suppose the white dot is now clockwise from the axis. You ask, ". . . and which is clearer now . . . this #5 . . . (pause, flip) . . . or #6?"
The pt chooses #5. Which way will you rotate the axis now?
a. Clockwise; go to 47e.
b. Counterclockwise; go to 48e.

47e

46e

−1.75 + 0.50 x 150
Yes. On choice #5 the white dot was clockwise to the axis. You realized that the pt had switched direction and is now heading back toward 120 degrees, where he or she started. What axis change would you choose now?
a. **−1.75 + 0.50 x 135**; go to 49e.
b. **−1.75 + 0.50 x 143**; go to 50e.

48e

46e

−1.75 + 0.50 x 150
No, you should follow the white dot from the position that the pt preferred.
Go back to 46e, and try again.

49e

47e

−1.75 + 0.50 x 135
No. We already tried axis 135 back in frame 44e. When the pt reverses direction, go back about halfway (about 7 degrees) between the last two choices.
Go back to 47e, and try again.

50e

47e

−1.75 + 0.50 x 143
Yes. You remembered that when the pt reverses direction that you should go back about halfway (about 7 degrees) between the last two choices. 143 is about halfway between 150 and 135.
Suppose the white dot is now counterclockwise to the axis. You ask, "Which seems best now? This #7 . . . or . . . (pause, flip) . . . #8 here?" The pt says they are about the same. What does this indicate?
a. The pt is not paying attention because one will always be better than the other; go to 51e.
b. You have reached the correct axis; go to 52e.

51e

50e

1.75 + 0.50 x 143
Oh, no! I hope you looked here out of mere curiosity and not because you really believe that choice a is correct!
Report back to frame 50e, and try again.

52e

50e

−1.75 + 0.50 x 143
Right! You remembered that when the two choices look the same that you have reached the end point. What should you do next?
a. Balance; go to 53e.
b. Turn the cross cyl so "P" aligns with the axis; go to 54e.

53e

52e

−1.75+ 0.50 x 143
No, you are not ready to balance yet. You have got to refine the cyl power first.
Go back to frame 52e, and try again.

54e

52e

−1.75 + 0.50 x 143
Yes, it is time to refine the cyl power. The chart is still on 20/80. The white dot is under the "P." (To help you keep your place, there is a (W) for white dot and an (R) for red so you know which dot is up on each choice.) You ask, "Which is the better now . . . #9(W) you are looking through here . . . (pause, flip) . . . or this #10(R)?" The pt chooses #9. What do you do now?
a. Add 0.25 cyl: **−1.75 + 0.75 x 143**; go to 55e.
b. Take out 0.25 cyl: **−1.75 + 0.25 x 143**; go to 56e.
c. Add 0.50 cyl: **−1.75 + 1.00 x 143**; go to 57e.
d. Take out 0.50 cyl: **−1.75 sph**; go to 58e.

55e

54e

−1.75 + 0.75 x 143
While you did remember to add plus cyl because the pt chose the lens that had the white dot showing, you forgot that cyl power refinement starts off in 0.50 steps.
Go back to 54e, and try again.

56e

54e

−1.75 + 0.25 x 143
No. Choice #9 had the white dot showing under the "P," indicating you should add more cyl.
Go back to 54e, and try again.

57e

54e

−1.75 + 1.00 x 143
Great! You realized that since the pt chose the lens with the white dot under "P" that you should add cyl. You also remembered to start offering 0.50-D steps. The red dot is now at "P." You ask, "Which is the clearer, this #11(R) . . . (pause, flip) . . . or #12(W)?" Pt chooses #12. Do you:
a. Add 0.50 cyl: **−1.75 + 1.50 x 143**; go to 59e.
b. Subtract 0.25 cyl: **−1.75 + 0.75 x 143**; go to 60e.

58e

54e

−1.75 sph
No. The pt chose #9, which had a white dot under the "P." This indicates that you should *add* cyl power. But at least you remembered to work in 0.50 steps!
Go back to 54e, and try again.

59e

57e

−1.75+ 1.50 x 143
Yes. Choice #12 had the white dot at "P." You continue refining power. What choice #s will you offer the pt next?
a. #13 and #14; go to 61e.
b. #1 and #2; go to 62e.

60e

57e

−1.75 + 0.75 x 143
No, choice #12 had the white dot showing, indicating the need for more cyl.
Go back to 57e, and try again.

61e

59e

−1.75 + 1.50 x 143
This is not wrong. But, it is a good idea to start back with #1 and #2 if the refractometry is prolonged.
Go on to frame 62e.

+

62e

59e, 61e

–1.75 + 1.50 x 143
Yes, it is a good idea to go back to saying #1
and #2 if the refractometry is prolonged.
(Using #13 and #14 is not wrong, of course.)
Suppose the pt took another 0.50 cyl:
–1.75 + 2.00 x 143
Now the red dot is on "P" and you ask, "Which
is clearer between these . . . this #1(R) . . .
(pause, flip) . . . or #2(W)?" The pt chooses #1.
Now you
a. Add another 0.50 cyl: **–1.75 + 2.50 x 143**; go
   to 63e.
b. Subtract 0.50 cyl: **–1.75 + 1.50 x 143**; go
   to 64e.
c. Subtract 0.25 cyl: **–1.75 + 1.75 x 143**; go
   to 65e.

63e

62e

–1.75 + 2.50 x 143
No, choice #1 had the red dot showing, indi-
cating you should reduce the cyl.
Go back to 62e, and try again.

64e

62e

–1.75 + 1.50 x 143
I am glad you remembered to reduce the
amount of cyl when the pt chooses a red dot at
"P." But you forgot to use 0.25 steps when the
pt reverses the pt's direction.
Go back to 62e, and try again.

65e

62e

–1.75 + 1.75 x 143
Wonderful! You remembered to reduce the cyl
power when the pt chooses a lens with the red
dot at "P." You also remembered to switch to
0.25 steps as soon as the pt reverses the pt's
direction. Now you should:
a. Have pt read the smallest letters possible; go
   to 66e.
b. Use the cross cyl one more time; go to 67e.
c. Move into fine spheres; go to 68e.

66e

65e

–1.75 + 1.75 x 143
No, you are jumping the gun but only by a fraction. You are not quite done with cyl power
refinement.
Go back to 65e, and try again.

67e

65e

–1.75 + 1.75 x 143
Right. You need to finish cyl power refinement.
The white dot is on "P"; and you ask, "Is this
#3(W) better . . . (pause, flip) . . . or this
#4(R)?" The pt chooses #3. Should you:
a. Give 0.25 cyl: **–1.75 + 2.00 x 143**; go to 69e.
b. Stay where you are; go to 70e.

68e

65e

–1.75 + 1.75 x 143
No, you are not quite done with cyl power
refinement.
Go back to 65e, and choose again.

69e

67e

–1.75 + 2.00 x 143
Although the pt did choose the lens with the
white dot at "P," remember that the pt was
already tested at +2.00 cyl back in frame 62e.
At that point, the pt requested less cyl, which
brought you to +1.75 cyl. The pt would probably flip–flop endlessly between +1.75 cyl and
+2.00 cyl.
Go back to 67e, and try again.

70e

67e

–1.75 + 1.75 x 143
Right. You remembered that the pt looked at
+2.00 cyl before and requested less power. The
pt might flip–flop forever between +2.00 cyl
and +1.75 cyl. You want to give the least
amount of cyl you can, so you use the +1.75
cyl and move the cross cylinder out of the way.
Next you should:
a. Move into fine spheres; go to 71e.
b. Have the pt read the smallest letters possible; go to 72e.

71e

70e

–1.75 + 1.75 x 143
No, not yet. How can you refine the sphere without a visual acuity reference from which to work?
Go back to 70e, and try again.

72e

70e

–1.75 + 1.75 x 143
Right. You need a visual acuity for a reference point when you start fine spheres. You have done a good job, and your pt now reads 20/25⁻. As you move into fine spheres, the acuity chart is set on:
a. 20/30; go to 73e.
b. 20/25; go to 74e.
c. 20/40; go to 75e

73e

72e

–1.75 + 1.75 x 143
Well, you already know the pt can read this. Refinement is better accomplished by trying to improve on the smallest letters that the pt can presently see.
Go to 72e, and choose again.

74e

72e

–1.75 + 1.75 x 143
Right. You want to refine from the smallest letters that the pt can see at this stage. You now switch to using spherical power and now should:
a. Offer +0.25: **–1.50 + 1.75 x 143**; go to 76e.
b. Offer –0.25: **–2.00 + 1.75 x 143**; go to 77e.

75e

72e

–1.75 + 1.75 x 143
No. You should refine from the smallest letters that the pt can recognize.
Return to 72e, and try again.

76e

74e

–1.50 + 1.75 x 143
Right! Always offer plus first. You also remembered that fine spheres works in 0.25-D steps. In this case, the pt says the letters have blurred a bit now. What next?
a. Return to **–1.75 + 1.75 x 143,** and quit; go to 78e.
b. Return to **–1.75 + 1.75 x 143,** and continue; go to 79e.

77e

74e

–2.00 + 1.75 x 143
No, always offer plus first.
Go to 74e, and choose again.

78e

76e

–1.75 + 1.75 x 143
No, you are not through! The +0.25 sph did not help, but you need to try a bit more minus now.
Go back to 76e, and try again.

79e

76e

–1.75 + 1.75 x 143
Right. Plus did not help; you need to try 0.25 minus sph next:
–2.00 + 1.75 x 143
The pt says the letters are clearer. Your next step is to:
a. Offer yet another –0.25: **–2.25 + 1.75 x 143** and ask if the letters got smaller; go to 80e.
b. Have the pt read the chart; go to 81e.

80e

79e

–2.25 + 1.75 x 143
While minification is a sign of over minusing, you forgot that a pt should be required to "earn" more minus by reading smaller letters on the chart before offering yet more minus.
Go to 79e, and choose again.

+

81e

79e

−2.00 + 1.75 x 143
Right! Always have the pt earn more minus by reading smaller letters. In this case, the pt now reads 20/25+. Now you should:
a. Offer another −0.25: **−2.25 + 1.75 x 143**; go to 82e.
b. Stop because this is adequate vision and such a big improvement over what you started with; go to 83e.

82e

81e

−2.25 + 1.75 x 143
Yes. But now you must require the pt to read smaller letters. And guess what? The pt reads 20/20! Congratulations!
Final MR: −2.25 + 1.75 x 143
VA **c** 20/20
Go to 84e.

83e

81e

−2.00 + 1.75 x 143
While this vision is a big improvement and certainly adequate, you should always try for 20/20.
Go back to 81e, and choose again.

84e
If you think you are worn out after working through this Exercise, just imagine how I felt after writing it! (It took six hours, plus two hours to type it!) You now have several options:
a. Rework this Exercise if you had difficulty with it; go to 1e.
b. Work another Exercise; go to Directory.

—

e. Unknown Refractive Error
MINUS CYLINDER

1e
NW: none
VA s̄ 20/200
Go to 2e.

2e

1e

Plano sph
You place the empty refractor to the pt. The chart is on:
a. 20/200; go to 3e.
b. 20/400; go to 4e.
c. 20/100; go to 5e.

3e

2e

Plano sph
No, it is better to start with letters a bit larger than the pt's starting acuity.
Go back to 2e, and try again.

4e

2e

Plano sph
Right. Ordinarily you would start at about 2 lines larger than the pt's starting acuity. But many charts do not have anything between 20/200 and 20/400. So 20/400 will have to do.
Go to 6e.

5e

2e

Plano sph
No, these are too small. You want to start with letters a bit larger than the pt's starting acuity.
Go back to 2e, and try again.

6e

4e

Plano sph
The pt affirms he or she can see the 20/400 letter. You are ready to start gross spheres. You first offer:
a. +0.25: **+0.25 sph**; go to 7e.
b. +0.50: **+0.50 sph**; go to 8e.
c. −0.50: **−0.50 sph**; go to 9e.

7e

6e

0.25 sph
Offering plus first is right, but gross spheres goes in 0.50-D steps, remember?
Go back to 6e, and try again.

8e

6e

+0.50 sph
Right! Gross spheres uses 0.50 steps, and you should always offer plus first. Next you should:
a. Add another 0.50: **+1.00 sph**; go to 10e.
b. Ask the pt if the chart is clearer; go to 11e.

9e

6e

−0.50 sph
No, always offer plus first.
Go back to 6e, and try again.

10e

8e

+1.00 sph
No, first you need to find out if the power change is helping or not.
Go back to 8e, and try again.

11e

8e

+0.50 sph
Yes, you should ask the pt if he or she notes any improvement after each plus change during gross spheres. In this case, the pt reports that the 20/400 letter is a bit clearer. Next you should:
a. Continue to add 0.50 steps of plus, assessing each change until the pt reports blurring; go to 12e.
b. Ask the pt how far down on the chart he or she can read now; go to 13e.

12e

11e

+0.50 sph
This is a good method for gross spheres . . . provided that the pt is taking plus. When the pt reports blurring, simply go 0.50 D back to the previous setting, then have the pt read the smallest letters possible.
Of course, this method is inappropriate when working in a minus direction, where the pt must 'earn' more minus by reading smaller letters.
Go to 14e.

13e

11e

+0.50 sph
There is nothing wrong with having the pt read the chart. But when adding plus it is quicker to move ahead in +0.50 steps until the pt reports blurring. At that point, simply go back 0.50 to the previous setting, then have the pt read the smallest letters possible.

Of course, this method is inappropriate when working in a minus direction.

Go to 14e.

14e

12e, 13e

+0.50 sph
After going through all that, let us suppose that the pt says that the letters are more blurred. You dutifully remove the +0.50:

Plano sph
Next you try giving:

a. –0.25: **–0.25 sph**; go to 15e.
b. –0.50: **–0.50 sph**; go to 16e.

15e

14e

–0.25 sph
No, gross spheres works in 0.50-D steps. Go back to 14e and try again.

16e

14e

–0.50 sph
Yes. You are still in gross spheres and using 0.50-D steps. The pt says this is clearer. Next you:

a. Offer another –0.50: **–1.00 sph**; go to 17e.
b. Have the pt read smaller letters; go to 18e.

17e

16e

–1.00 sph
Well, while it is true that a 0.50-D step probably will not take the pt from 20/200 to 20/20, it is best to be cautious when offering minus.

Go back to 16e, and choose again.

18e

16e

–0.50 sph
Right. When the pt takes minus, the pt should earn it by reading smaller letters with each change.

Go to 19e.

19e

18e

–0.50 sph
Let us suppose that the pt says that the 20/200 is clearer, but the pt still cannot read 20/100. Next you should:

a. Check for astigmatism; go to 20e.
b. Offer more minus; go to 21e.

20e

19e

–0.50 sph
No, you are jumping the gun a bit. Although this may be the most minus the pt should have, you should offer more minus this time because the pt's acuity is still so poor. The next 0.50 change may yield 20/100.

Go back to 19e, and choose again.

21e

19e

–0.50 sph
Yes, you should offer more minus. The pt's poor acuity may take a substantial amount of minus to improve it. So you try another –0.50:

–1.00 sph
and the pt reads 20/100. In fact, you continue in –0.50 steps, and the pt reads smaller letters each time for TWO more steps:

–2.00 sph
Now the pt reads 20/60. You give another –0.50:

–2.50 sph
The pt says this is better, but still reads only 20/60.

Next you:

a. Go back 0.50: **–2.00 sph**; go to 22e.
b. Offer another –0.50: **–3.00 sph**; go to 23e.

22e

21e

–2.00 sph
This is fine. You are sure you have not over minused this way. If the pt needs more minus, the pt will pick it up in fine spheres. (The other choice was okay, too.) You are ready to check for astigmatism.

Go to 26e.

23e

21e

–3.00 sph
This is fine. (The other choice was okay, too.)
In this case, the pt still cannot read more than
20/60. Now you should return to:
a. **–2.50 sph**; go to 24e.
b. **–2.00 sph**; go to 25e.

24e

23e

–2.50 sph
No, you did not go back far enough. The last
TWO changes (a total of 1.00) did not produce
any improvement, and you want the least
minus possible.
Go back to 23e, and choose again.

25e

23e

–2.00 sph
Right. The last TWO changes (a total of 1.00)
did not produce any improvement, and you
want the least minus possible. You are now
ready to check for astigmatism.
Go to 26e.

26e

22e, 25e

–2.00 sph
You are going to use the astigmatic dial to
detect astigmatism. You show the pt the dial
and ask:
a. Are there any lines that are darker than the
   rest? Go to 27e.
b. Are any of the lines more blurred than the
   rest? Go to 28e.

27e

26e

–2.00 sph
Right. You need to know if there are darker
lines. If the pt says all the lines look the same,
what do you do next?
a. Go directly to fine spheres; go to 29e.
b. Add +0.50: **–1.50 sph**; go to 30e.

28e

26e

–2.00 sph
No, you need to identify the darker lines.
Go back to 26e, and try again.

29e

27e

–2.00 sph
No, you are not ready for fine spheres yet. If all
the lines look the same, add 0.50 of plus:
–1.50 sph
If astigmatism is present, this maneuver will
usually make it apparent.
Go to 30e.

30e

27e, 29e

–1.50 sph
Right. The addition of 0.50 of plus sph will
often bring out the darker lines. Suppose the pt
now says that the lines running from 10 o'clock
across to 4 o'clock are darker. Where do you set
your axis?
a. 060 degrees; go to 31e.
b. 120 degrees; go to 32e.

31e

30e

–1.50 –   x 060
No, you need to review the "rule of 30."
Go back to 30e, and choose again.

32e

30e

–1.50 –   x 120
Right. Using the "rule of 30," multiply the
smaller clock hour by 30. In this case,
4 o'clock is smaller; 4 x 30 = 120. Your next
step is to:
a. Add cyl power until all lines seem equal; go
   to 33e.
b. Go back to the eye chart, flip down the cross
   cyl, and get busy; go to 34e.

33e

32e

–1.50 –   x 120
Right. Now, suppose the lines seem equal after
0.50 D of cyl is given:
–1.50 – 0.50 x 120
Next you should:
a. Remove the 0.50 of plus sph you used to
   identify the astigmatism: **–2.00 – 0.50 x 120**;
   go to 35e.
b. Give +0.25 sphere power for each –0.50 D
   of cyl power you used: **–1.25 – 0.50 x 120**;
   go to 36e.

34e

32e

–1.50 –   x 120
No, not yet. You need to determine about how
much cyl power the pt needs.
Go back to 32e, and try again.

35e

33e

–2.00 – 0.50 x 120
No. You need to adjust the sphere according to
how much cyl you used.
Go back to 33e, and choose again.

36e

33e

–1.25 – 0.50 x 120
Right! Go to 37e.

37e

36e

–1.25 – 0.50 x 120
Now you are ready to return to the letter chart.
What size letters do you choose to begin the
cross cyl stage? (Last acuity was 20/60.)
a. 20/80; go to 38e.
b. 20/60; go to 39e.
c. 20/40; go to 40e.

38e

37e

–1.25 – 0.50 x 120
Right. The 20/80 line is two lines above the acuity after gross spheres. During cross cyl refinement, you want to use letters that you know the
pt can see. Now, you pop the cross cyl into
place. How do you line it up to check the axis?
a "P" in line with the axis; go to 41e.
b. Turnstile in line with axis; go to 42e.

39e

37e

–1.25 – 0.50 x 120
No. 20/60 is the pt's acuity after gross spheres.
You need something easier to see.
Go back to 37e, and choose again.

40e

37e

–1.25 – 0.50 x 120
No. This is even smaller than the pt's acuity
after gross spheres. You need letters that the pt
can see easily.
Go back to 37e, and choose again.

41e

38e

–1.25 – 0.50 x 120
No, the "P" is for power refinement.
Go back to 38e, and try again.

42e

38e

–1.25 – 0.50 x 120
Yes. The turnstile is aligned with the axis when
you refine axis position. Suppose the red dot is
clockwise to your 120 degree axis. You now
ask, "Which is clearer, this #1. . . (pause, flip)
. . . or #2?" The pt says #2 is clearer. Which
way do you rotate the axis now?
a. Clockwise 15 degrees: **–1.25 – 0.50 x 105**;
   go to 43e.
b. Counterclockwise 15 degrees: **–1.25 – 0.50
   x 135**; go to 44e.

43e

42e

–1.25 – 0.50 x 105
No, you should follow the red dot. When you
flipped the cross cyl over for choice #2, this
placed the red dot counterclockwise from the
turnstile.
Go back to 42e, and try again.

44e

42e

–1.25 – 0.50 x 135
Right. You realized that flipping the cross cyl over for choice #2 placed the red dot counterclockwise to the turnstile, where it remains.
You now say, "And now which seems better, this #3 . . . (pause, flip) . . . or #4?" The pt chooses #3. Where do you rotate the axis now?
a. Clockwise 15 degrees: **–1.25 – 0.50 X 120**, go to 45e.
b. Counterclockwise 15 degrees:
   –1.25 – 0.50 x 160; go to 46e.

45e

44e

–1.25 – 0.50 x 120
No. The pt chose #3, which had the red dot in a counterclockwise direction. You should follow the red dot.
Reread frame 44e, and choose again.

46e

44e

–1.25 – 0.50 x 150
Yes. During choice #3, the red dot was counterclockwise from the turnstile. Following the red dot 15 degrees counterclockwise brought you to 150 degrees. Suppose the red dot is now clockwise from the axis. You ask, "Which is clearer now . . . this #5 . . . (pause, flip) . . . or #6?"
The pt chooses #5. Which way will you rotate the axis now?
a. Clockwise; go to 47e.
b. Counterclockwise; go to 48e.

47e

46e

–1.25 – 0.50 x 160
Yes. On choice #5 the red dot was clockwise to the axis. You realized that the pt had switched direction, and the pt is now heading back toward 120 degrees. where the pt started. What axis change would you choose now?
a. **–1.25 – 0.50 x 135**; go to 49e.
b. **–1.25 – 0.50 x 143**; go to 50e.

48e

46e

–1.25 – 0.50 x 150
No, you should follow the red dot from the position that the pt preferred.
Go back to 46e, and try again.

49e

47e

–1.25 – 0.50 x 135
No. We already tried axis 135 back in frame 44e. When the pt reverses direction, go back about halfway (about 7 degrees) between the last two choices.
Go back to 47e, and try again.

50e

47e

–1.25 – 0.50 x 143
Yes. You remembered that when the pt reverses direction, you should go back about halfway (about 7 degrees) between the last two choices. 143 is about halfway between 150 and 135. Suppose the red dot is now counterclockwise to the axis. You ask, "Which seems better now? This #7 . . . or . . . (pause, flip) . . .#8 here?" The pt says they are about the same. What does this indicate?
a. The pt is not paying attention because one will always be better than the other; go to 51e.
b. You have reached the correct axis; go to 52e.

51e

50e

–1.25 – 0.50 x 143
Oh, no! I hope you looked here out of mere curiosity and not because you really believe that choice a is correct.
Report back to frame 50e, and try again.

52e

50e

–1.25 – 0.50 x 143
Right! You remembered that when the two choices look the same that you have reached the end point. What should you do next?
a. Balance; go to 53e
b. Turn the cross cyl so "P" aligns with the axis; go to 54e.

53e

52e

–1.25 – 0.50 x 143

No, you are not ready to balance yet. You have got to refine the cyl power first.

Go back to frame 52e, and try again.

54e

52e

–1.25 – 0.50 x 143

Yes, it is time to refine the cyl power. The chart is still on 20/80. The red dot is under the "P." (To help you keep your place, there is a (W) for white and an (R) for red so you know which dot is up on each choice.) You ask, "Which is the better now . . . #9(R) you are looking through here . . . (pause, flip) . . . or this #10(W)?"

The pt chooses #9. What do you do now?

a. Give 0.25 cyl: **–1.25 – 0.75 x 143**; go to 55e.

b. Take out 0.25 cyl: **–1.25 – 0.25 x 143**; go to 56e.

c. Give 0.50 cyl: **–1.25 – 1.00 x 143**; go to 57e.

d. Take out 0.50 cyl: **–1.25 sph**; go to 58e.

55e

54e

–1.25 – 0.75 x 143

While you did remember to add minus cyl because the pt chose the lens that had the red dot showing, you forgot that cyl power refinement starts off in 0.50 steps.

Go back to 54e, and try again.

56e

54e

–1.25 – 0.25 x 143

No. Choice #9 had the red dot showing under the "P," indicating you should give more cyl.

Go back to 54e, and try again.

57e

54e

–1.25 – 1.00 x 143

Great! You realized that since the pt chose the lens with the red dot under "P," you should give cyl. You also remembered to use 0.50-D steps. The white dot is now at "P." You ask, "Which is clearer, this #11(W) . . . (pause, flip) . . . or #12(R)? Pt chooses #12. Do you:

a. Give 0.50 cyl: **–1.25 – 1.50 x 143**; go to 59e.

b. Remove 0.25 cyl: **–1.25 – 0.75 x 143**; go to 60e.

58e

54e

–1.25 sph

No. The pt chose #9, which had a red dot under the "P." This indicates that you should give cyl power. But at least you remembered to work in 0.50 steps!

Go back to 54e, and try again.

59e

57e

–1.25 – 1.50 x 143

Yes. Choice #12 had the red dot at "P." You continue refining power. What choice #s will you offer the pt next?

a. #13 and #14; go to 61e.

b. #1 and #2; go to 62e.

60e

57e

–1.25 – 0.75 x 143

No, choice #12 had the red dot showing, indicating the need for more cyl.

Go back to 57e, and try again.

61e

59e

–1.25 – 1.50 x 143

This is not wrong. But it is a good idea to start back with #1 and #2 if the refractometry is prolonged.

Go on to frame 62e.

62e

59e, 61e

–1.25 – 1.50 x 143

Yes, it is a good idea to go back to saying #1 and #2 if the refractometry is prolonged. (Using #13 and #14 is not wrong, of course.) Suppose the pt took another 0.50 cyl:

–1.25 – 2.00 x 143

Now the white dot is on "P," and you ask, "Which is clearer between these . . . this #1(W) . . . (pause, flip) . . . or #2(R)?" The pt chooses #1. Now you:

a. Give 0.50 cyl: **–1.25 – 2.50 x 143**; go to 63e.

b. Remove 0.50 cyl: **–1.25 – 1.50 x 143**; go to 64e.

c. Remove 0.25 cyl: **–1.25 – 1.75 x 143**; go to 65e.

63e

62e

1.25 – 2.50 x 143

No, choice #1 had the white dot showing, indicating you should reduce the cyl.
Go back to 62e, and try again.

64e

62e

–1.25 – 1.50 x 143

I am glad you remembered to reduce the amount of cyl when the pt chooses a white dot at "P." But you forgot to use 0.25 steps when the pt reverses the pt's direction.
Go back to 62e, and try again.

65e

62e

–1.25 – 1.75 x 143

Wonderful! You remembered to reduce the cyl power when the pt chooses a lens with the white dot at "P." You also remembered to switch to 0.25 steps as soon as the pt reverses the pt's direction. Now you should
a. Have pt read smallest letters possible; go to 66e.
b. Use the cross cyl one more time; go to 67e.
c. Move into fine spheres; go to 68e.

66e

65e

–1.25 – 1.75 x 143

No, you are jumping the gun, but only by a fraction. You are not quite done with cyl power refinement.
Go back to 65e, and try again.

67e

65e

–1.25 – 1.75 x 143

Right. You need to finish cyl power refinement. The red dot is on "P," and you ask, "Is this #3(R) the better . . . (pause, flip) . . . or this #4(W)?" The pt chooses #3. Should you:
a. Give 0.25 cyl: **–1.25 – 2.00 x 143**; go to 69e.
b. Stay where you are; go to 70e.

68e

65e

–1.25 – 1.75 x 143

No, you are not quite done with cyl power refinement.
Go back to 65e, and choose again.

69e

67e

–1.25 – 2.00 x 143

Although the pt did choose the lens with the red dot at "P," remember that the pt was already tested at –2.00 cyl back in frame 62e. At that point, the pt requested less cyl, which brought you to –1.75 cyl. The pt would probably flip–flop endlessly between –1.75 cyl and –2.00 cyl.
Go back to 67e, and try again.

70e

67e

–1.25 – 1.75 x 143

Right. You remembered that the pt looked at –2.00 cyl before and requested less power. The pt might flip–flop forever between –2.00 cyl and –1.75 cyl. You want to give the least amount of cyl you can, so you use the –1.75 cyl and move the cross cylinder out of the way. Next you should:
a. Move into fine spheres; go to 71e.
b. Have the pt read the smallest letters possible; go to 72e.

71e

70e

–1.25 – 1.75 x 143

No, not yet. How can you refine the sphere without a visual acuity reference from which to work?
Go back to 70e, and try again.

72e

70e

–1.25 – 1.75 x 143

Right. You need a visual acuity for a reference point when you start fine spheres. You have done a good job, and your pt now reads 20/25⁻. As you move into fine spheres, the acuity chart is set on:
a. 20/30; go to 73e.
b. 20/25; go to 74e.
c. 20/40; go to 75e

73e

72e

–1.25 – 1.75 x 143
Well, you already know the pt can read this. Refinement is better accomplished by trying to improve on the smallest letters that the pt can presently see.
Go to 72e, and choose again.

74e

72e

–1.25 – 1.75 x 143
Right. You want to refine from the smallest letters that the pt can see at this stage. You now switch to using spherical power and now should:
a. Offer +0.25: **–1.00 – 1.75 x 143**; go to 76e.
b. Offer –0.25: **–1.50 – 1.75 x 143**; go to 77e.

75e

72e

–1.25 – 1.75 x 143
No. You should refine from the smallest letters that the pt can recognize.
Return to 72e, and try again.

76e

74e

–1.00 – 1.75 x 148
Right! Always offer plus first. You also remembered that fine spheres works in 0.25-D steps. In this case, the pt says the letters have blurred a bit now. What next?
a. Return to **–1.25 – 1.75 x 143,** and quit; go to 78e
b. Return to **–1.25 – 1.75 x 143,** and continue; go to 79e.

77e

74e

–1.50 – 1.75 x 143
No, always offer plus first.
Go to 74e, and choose again.

78e

76e

–1.25 – 1.75 x 143
No, you are not through! The +0.25 sph did not help, but you need to try a bit more minus now.
Go back to 76e, and try again.

79e

76e

–1.25 – 1.75 x 143
Right. Plus did not help, you need to try 0.25 minus sph next:
–1.50 – 1.75 x 143
The pt says the letters are clearer. Your next step is to:
a. Offer yet another –0.25: **–1.75 – 1.75 x 143** and ask if the letters got smaller; go to 80e.
b. Have the pt read the chart; go to 81e.

80e

79e

–1.75 – 1.75 x 143
While minification is a sign of over minusing, you forgot that a pt should be required to "earn" more minus by reading smaller letters on the chart before offering yet more minus.
Go to 79e, and choose again.

81e

79e

–1.50 – 1.75 x 143
Right! Always have the pt earn more minus by reading smaller letters. In this case, the pt now reads 20/25+. Now you should:
a. Offer another –0.25: **–1.75 – 1.75 x 143**, go to 82e.
b. Stop, because this is adequate vision and such a big improvement over what you started with; go to 83e.

82e

81e

–1.75 – 1.75 x 143
Yes. But now you must require the pt to read smaller letters. And guess what? The pt reads 20/20! Congratulations!
Final MR: –1.75 – 1.75 x 143
VA c̄ 20/20
Go to 84e.

83e

81e

–1.50 – 1.75 x 143
While this vision is a big improvement and certainly adequate, you should always try for 20/20.
Go back to 81e, and choose again.

84e
If you think you are worn out after working through this Exercise, just imagine how I felt after writing it! (It took six hours, plus two hours to type it, plus one hour to reverse it to minus cyl!) You now have several options:
a. Rework this Exercise if you had difficulty with it; go to 1e.
b. Work another Exercise; go to Directory.

Index